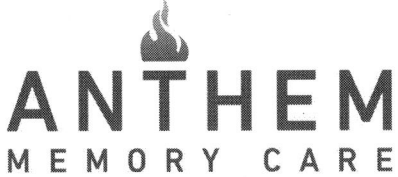

This book is dedicated to all who belong to the Anthem Family.

Anthem Memory Care is a community — and a family.

Anthem Memory Care Communities provide highly specialized care for individuals affected by dementia — including Alzheimer's Disease, Lewy Bodies, Fronto-Temporal, Vascular, Parkinson, and Huntington..

Each Anthem Community has been strategically tailored to meet the unique needs of our residents. Our goal is to enrich the lives of every resident and offer peace of mind to family members by focusing on individual, person-centered care.

We seek to inspire significance and convey understanding to our residents and their families. Meaningful engagement plays a key role in the quality of every Anthem resident's life. *Pathways of Purpose*, our proprietary life-engagement program, offers a tailored approach to activities that affirms each individual's identity and creates opportunities for connections within the community. It supports well-being by affirming identity, facilitating connections with others, recognizing autonomy, promoting feelings of security, and offering events and activities that celebrate joyful living.

We all need a sense of purpose — goals, direction, and a feeling that our lives have meaning. It's crucial to our well-being, and a dementia diagnosis does not change this basic need. Anthem ensures that residents live well despite living with dementia. Our philosophy of engagement is rooted in trusted relationships, compassion, empathy, empowering, support, and *doing with* rather than *doing for*. It focuses on resident strengths and minimizes disabilities in order to promote feelings of autonomy, competence, success, and pleasure.

As you read this book by dementia expert Dr. Tam Cummings, your knowledge of the nine common dementias will increase, and you will gain valuable insights that will enable you to interact with your loved one with less stress and greater joy. As we travel this journey together, rest assured we accept you and the other members of your family as trusted partners in providing the best care possible for your loved one.

Copyright © 2022 Tam Cummings. All Rights Reserved. Published in the United States by The Dementia Association LLC. All rights reserved.
Printed in the United States of America.
No part of this book, either in its published or electronic format, may be reproduced in any manner whatsoever, stored in a retrieval system, distributed or transmitted in any form or by any means, including electronic, mechanical, photocopying, recording, scanning or otherwise, without the prior written permission of the publisher, except in the case of brief quotations embodied in critical articles and reviews and certain other noncommercial uses permitted by copyright law. For permission requests, email the Publisher via The Dementia Association LLC or TamCummings.com.

Cummings, Tam, 1961-
The Itty Bitty Dementia, Tam Cummings, PhD – 1st edition
ISBN: 099096373X
ISBN: 9798398335743 (soft cover)
1.Dementia. 2. Alzheimer's Disease. 3. Health Education. 4. Aging. 5. Mental Health
First Edition
10 9 8 7 6 5 4 3

Dedication

Wilma Jean Smith Sargent
1921-2020
My other Mother.
She kept me safe. She taught me faith.
A wise and truly funny lady.
Godspeed my dear friend.

Contents

CHAPTER ONE: DEMENTIA IS A BRAIN DISEASE 1

CHAPTER TWO: THE BRAIN'S LOBES 21

CHAPTER THREE: WHAT IS MEMORY? 31

CHAPTER FOUR: THE NINE MOST COMMON DEMENTIAS 56

CHAPTER FIVE: STAGING DEMENTIA 96

One
DEMENTIA IS A BRAIN DISEASE

Dementia caregivers are often challenged to understand the disease and its impact on themselves and their loved one. Information about these brain diseases is confusing. Medical professionals are often uninformed about the many types of dementia, the disease process, and the extent of the damage to the brain.

Rather than addressing dementias with a medical approach, the lack of research, understanding and education means that care for your loved one is not always coherent, consistent, or rooted in causation. Some caregivers seem innately aware of the mental and physical decline that Persons with Dementia (PWD) experience, while others have difficulty separating the disease from the person.

The lack of general knowledge about the progression of dementias is also hampered by how People with Dementia appear throughout most of the disease process. People with Dementia typically do not seem physically ill until the final stages of the disease. It is only after significant brain tissue loss that the

Why Do We Need to Understand Dementia?

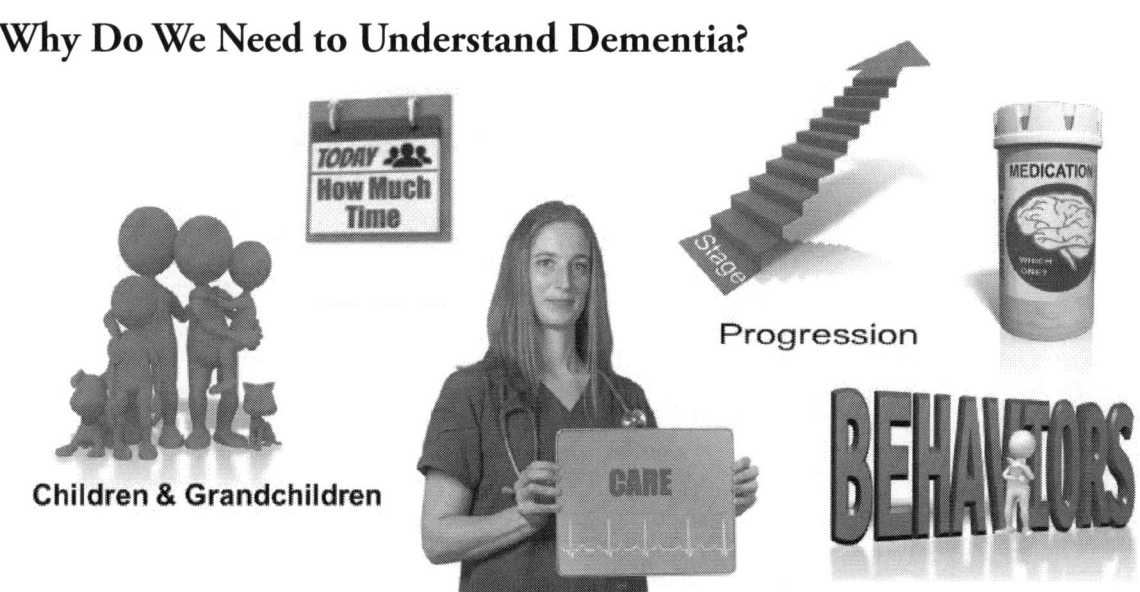

illness becomes apparent — in their posture, facial features, and amid moments of apparent confusion. You may witness weight loss or a lack of facial or vocal emotion. They may speak in monotones, use a shuffling gait, lose some aspects of language, experience a decline in executive function, and display an inability to perform coordinated movements like chewing food and swallowing.

These are some of the outward physical changes caregivers may witness. These symptoms arise after the brain loses a significant one pound or more of cells and tissue. Only then will the Person with Dementia begin to look sick to outsiders and professionals.

Dementia is one of the most confusing medical words we encounter. Its original translation from French means incapacitation of the mental faculties. But that translation never made it to today's interpretation. Instead, families and many professionals think dementia is the name of an illness affecting memory. It is not.

Five Questions All Families Need to Ask

Dementia is the umbrella term for a group of brain diseases. It is not the name of a particular form, although it may be the term the doctor uses until a definitive diagnosis is made. Diagnosing the type of dementia or dementias in your loved one may require more than two dozen medical tests, including blood work, a spinal tap, EEG, EKG, MRI, and cognitive measurements. The testing requires a specialist, like a neurologist who focuses on dementias, to review the tests. The doctor will also include personal observations of the person as well as input from the family in making a final diagnosis.

Think of dementias the way you have been taught to think about cancer. Cancer is also an umbrella term. Cancer means malignant cells are attacking the body. There are more than 400 identified cancers, and cancers have domains or subsets. Isn't it common to ask which breast cancer form? Which skin cancer form? Which bone cancer form?

Likewise, it is critical that the form of dementia be diagnosed, just as we expect the type of cancer to be diagnosed. The diagnosis considers the family's health history. The type of dementia determines its progression, behaviors, medications, and how to plan care.

Question 1: Which Dementia Does Your Loved One Have?

Dementia is the umbrella term for a group of diseases affecting the brain. The disease impacts at least two of the seven lobes of the brain. It is progressive, meaning the person cannot recover or regain abilities. It interferes with the ability to function or complete the Activities of daily living (ADLs). Activities of daily Living include the ability to transfer, walk, toilet, bathe, groom, dress, and eat. Dementia interferes with memory.

Memory is required for the activities of daily living, plus language, unassisted movement, balance, and the recognition of self and others. Memory is everything we are able to do in life.

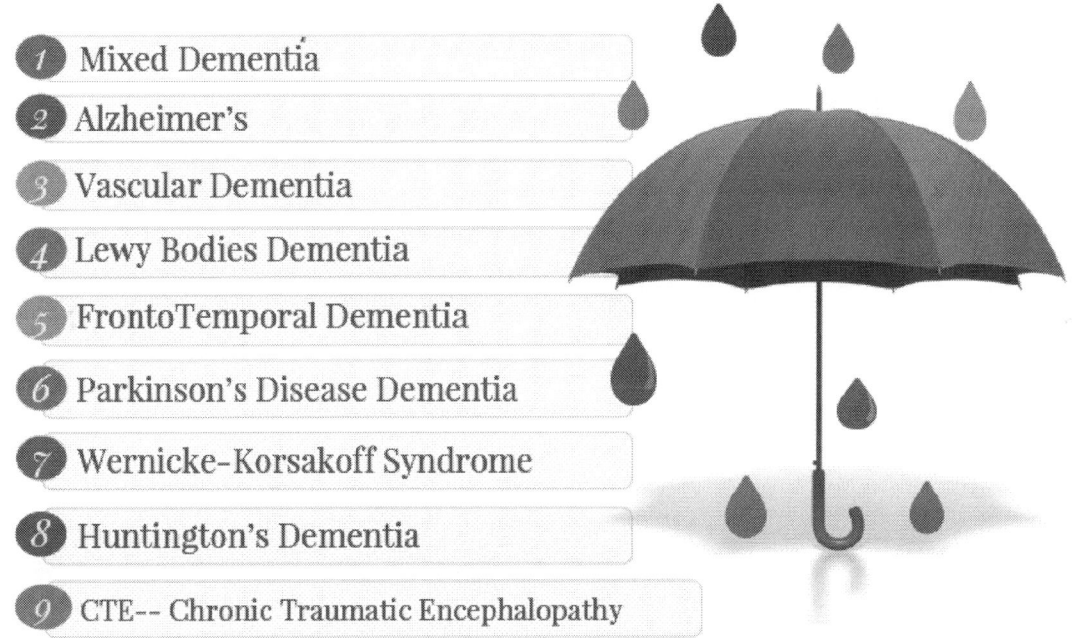

Nine Most Common Dementias

1. Mixed Dementia
2. Alzheimer's
3. Vascular Dementia
4. Lewy Bodies Dementia
5. FrontoTemporal Dementia
6. Parkinson's Disease Dementia
7. Wernicke-Korsakoff Syndrome
8. Huntington's Dementia
9. CTE-- Chronic Traumatic Encephalopathy

The type of dementia also determines the types of behaviors a Person with Dementia might display. Some dementias include sexual behaviors, such as a heightened interest in sex or inappropriate comments about sexual activity. Others might display scatological (feces) behaviors. Some dementias include sudden outbursts of crying or laughing without any apparent cause. Other dementias cause people to overeat, while still other dementias mean the person is prone to anorexia.

Some of the dementias attack the brain aggressively. Generally, the younger a person is, the more aggressively the dementia damages the brain. Other dementias can linger for decades in the brain with no noticeable ill effects, awaiting some silent signal to begin the destruction caused by the failure of proteins in the brain tissue.

The type of dementia also dictates medication usage. Some medications slow the disease progression by allowing a chemical connection between brain cells to work a bit longer. Other medications stop the buildup of glutamate in the cells.

Dementia is defined by seven progressive stages. One group of medications works best in the early part of the disease — in Stages Two (also called Mild Cognitive Impairment or MCI) — or to persons in Stages Three or Four.

Unfortunately, most persons are not diagnosed until the late or terminal stages. The dementia diagnosis is generally made in Stage Five. In this stage there is significant brain tissue damage although the person will not yet appear physically ill.

Medications may slow the progression of the disease during the worst stages, when the person has suffered significant brain damage and is no longer herself. Physicians may neglect to discuss with families the risks and benefits of medications during later stages of the disease.

Many medical professionals fail to discuss these important issues with the family caregiver. Would the Person with Dementia want medication that extends the disease during these difficult final stages of significant brain tissue loss? Would she want her caregiver to literally kill himself providing care or spend the sum of a life's savings for final care and leave the caregiver penniless? Would she simply prefer to be kept comfortable during the final stages of a terminal illness?

The type of dementia also indicates heredity or sporadic genetic assignment. Huntington's Dementias are hereditary. Early Onset Familial Alzheimer's Dementia is hereditary. And since forms of vascular disease are hereditary, so the forms of dementia caused by vascular disease would also follow. The type of dementia tells

NOTES

the caregiver how much time is left. From very aggressive to very slow, different forms of dementia advance in their own way. Staging the Person with Dementia every two to three months allows caregivers to track the decline, the behaviors, and prepare for the next stages of the disease.

The type of dementia will begin to answer the questions about what kind of care your loved one needs. Some communities are simply not large enough or skilled enough to provide care for some types of behavioral dementias.

Question 2: Do You Understand the Brain is Dying?

In basic brain function, one cell gathers an electrical charge and the neurotransmitters (chemicals in the brain) fire a signal down a dendrite (root), across a space to the next cell. When the neurotransmitter is received, the new cell releases a chemical, signaling enzymes to move into the space and eat or clear the pathway of used up neurotransmitter parts and pieces.

As proteins begin to break apart in the brain fluid between the cells, the resulting plaque is thought to trigger a reaction of the tau proteins in the dendrites (roots) of the cells. The tau protein begins to break apart, to curl and tangle, causing the dendrites to tangle as well. The space between cells slowly stretches farther apart as the roots shrivel.

Normally, the first cell fires its electrical charge sending neurotransmitters across the cell, through the dendrites, firing across the synapse (space) to the next cell. This second cell receives the neurotransmitters into docking spaces and the connection repeats to the next cell. Then enzymes sweep across the synapse to clear the debris for the cell's next function.

Starving neurons from folding Tau

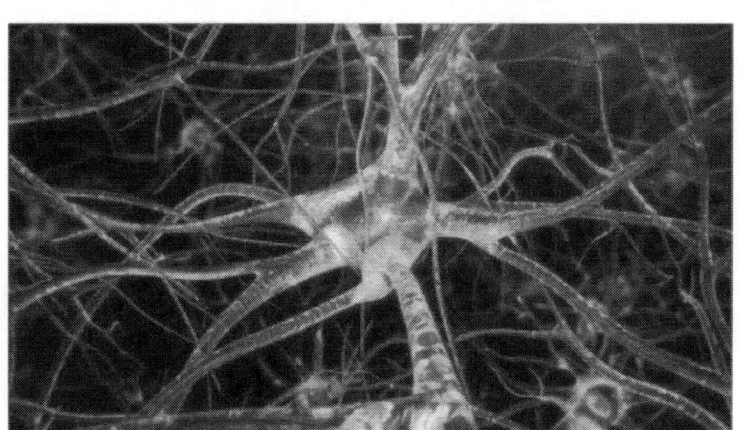

As the cell begins to

shrivel, it continues to attempt to function. But the neurotransmitter can't get through to the next cell because the synapse is now a bit farther away. As the first cell fires its charge, the enzymes wait and attack as though the cells are functioning normally and are still close to each other.

Some dementia medications cause a reaction in the cell function that allows the connection between the cells to work longer. They remain effective until there is too much space between the cells, or the cell has finally starved. Once dead, the cell is removed, and the space gets refilled with cerebral spinal fluid. In most forms of dementia, the brain cells starve, die, and are removed from the brain as waste.

At night, when we reach deep sleep, our brains cells draw up to allow the brain to wash itself clean of broken bits and pieces of cells and proteins. That's why you wake up refreshed and clear-headed for the next day.

Brain cells also die from a lack of oxygen caused by some form of vascular event. Strokes, for example, interrupt blood flow to areas of the brain. The specific lobe affected by the suddenly dead or damaged brain cells causes the Person with Dementia to behave differently. Where those cells once existed, the space is now filled with cerebral spinal fluid. Bit by bit, cell by cell, the brain is destroyed.

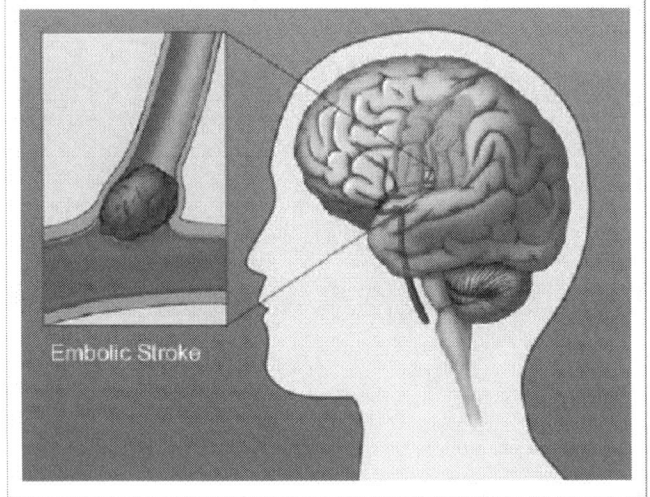

Strokes stop blood supply to cells

Oddly enough, even as the brain is dying, it is only when a pound of tissue is compromised that a loved one will begin to appear physically different. Eventually, the cranium containing a three-pound brain will have more spinal-fluid weight than brain-cell weight.

In the beginning, this person's brain was like yours or mine, an amazing collection of 100 billion neurons doing trillions of activities per second. The

Brain Comparison

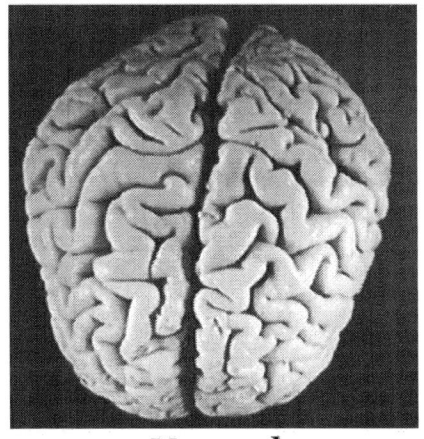
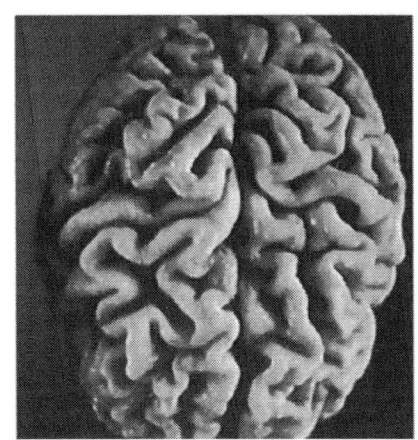

Ilustración: North Carolina Alzheimer's Association

Normal *vs* Alzheimer's

brain retrieves and stores information, allowing growth, learning, and life. Using electrical charges and a variety of neurotransmitters (chemicals in the brain), the brain continues to try to function even when it has only a pound or so of remaining tissue. It is the most complex and impressive organ in the human body.

The sheer number of brain cells and connections helps to explain why sudden resurgences of cognition and conversation can occur after months of silence and/or forgetfulness. The brain continues seeking pathways, even when heavily damaged. A sudden rush or release of these neurotransmitter chemicals may occur from excitement, sudden noise, movement, or even increased socialization. That sudden resurgence can make you believe your loved one's brain has improved or recovered.

As the form of dementia progresses and more and more brain cells slowly die, the operation and interpretation of electrical signals is interrupted or lost. As increasing numbers of cells die, the Person with Dementia is less able to control her body, which the brain also runs.

Over time, the Person with Dementia loses the brain cells that hold information and instructions for the Instrumental Activities of Daily Living (IADLS), including independent living, managing money, shopping for and preparing food, operating a television, telephone, or computer, performing housework and laundry, taking medications, and managing transportation.

During this period of change, the decline in a person's ability to perform the

Activities of Daily Living (ADLs) — including transferring, walking, toileting, bathing, dressing, grooming, and eating — proceeds in a steady and relentless manner. There are fewer brain cells operating correctly with each passing day.

In Vascular Dementias, the vascular causes can be addressed medically, but even with medical intervention, the decline continues. Brain cells continue to die, resulting in continued damage and decline. Eventually, as with all dementias, there won't be enough brain cells to maintain life.

Providing care at the beginning of symptoms typically requires 10 years or more at home, before the person requires professional care. Early care needs to include verbal reminders, notes, calendars, and increasing explanations for each of the steps related to the activities of daily living and instrumental activities of daily living. As the dementia progresses, the family caregiver may be performing all the instrumental activities and assisting the person with daily living activities.

Question 3: Has Your Loved One Started Falling Yet?

Most human behavior involves using the motor and movement areas of the brain. Whether it's talking, eating, gesturing, driving, texting, bathing, dressing, etc., movement is constant. If the motor cortex becomes damaged, any individual would be challenged or even unable to successfully begin and complete movement.

This includes coordinated movements and motor functions, as well as

Dementia falls are expected

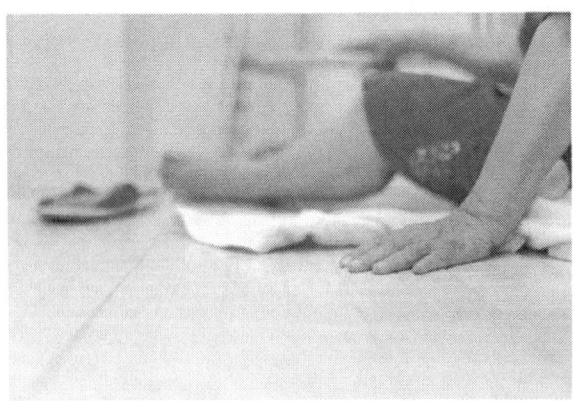

1. Mixed Dementia
2. Alzheimer's—back into chair
3. Vascular Dementia—face, knees, elbows
4. Lewy Bodies Dementia—stiff forward/back
5. FrontoTemporal Dementia—bent at waist
6. Parkinson's Disease Dementia—LBD
7. Wernicke-Korsakoff Syndrome
8. Huntington's Dementias
9. CTE-- Chronic Traumatic Encephalopathy

the memory required to perform each step of the activities of daily living. Unfortunately, a damaged brain also leads to falls. The falls experienced by People with Dementia are directly related to a change in both coordination and perception due to brain damage. The slow and gradual destruction of the four areas located at the top of the brain means the Person with Dementia eventually will not be capable of movement.

The damage and loss of the primary motor cortex, the premotor cortex, the supplementary motor cortex, and the posterior parietal cortex renders the Person with Dementia unable to move parts of their body. Walking, eating, and holding the head erect will all be affected as the dementia progresses.

These areas of the brain are the first to display signs of the disease in most forms of dementia. In the beginning, the cortexes experience slight damage. Enough healthy brain structure allows the person to continue to function, but eventually the motor areas are completely destroyed. People with Dementia in Stage Seven of the disease become bed-bound and totally reliant upon others for care due to extensive brain damage. Your loved one isn't reluctant to try to move; she simply can't due to brain damage.

Alzheimer's Dementias begin in the four cortexes, leading to early stumbles or missteps. It only takes a slight change in coordination, a subtle variance in lifting the foot properly, to create a fall. All other movement is being affected as well, but we are less likely to notice subtle changes in chewing, eye and hand coordination, driving, dressing, or bringing food or drink to the mouth.

Brain damage from each form of dementia makes falls an expected event. Falls are a symptom, a sign of the disease. Falls are not a sign of poor care; they are a sign of specific brain damage caused by dementia. Unfortunately, regulatory agencies and medical providers are not always aware that brain damage equals functional impairment in People with Dementia. Medical professionals and families must plan for and anticipate falls and prepare for the coming decline.

Destruction of brain tissue causes other problems. Normal aging can include the gradual loss of peripheral vision, which allows you to see to the side while

NOTES

Care Plan: Broken Hips are Coming

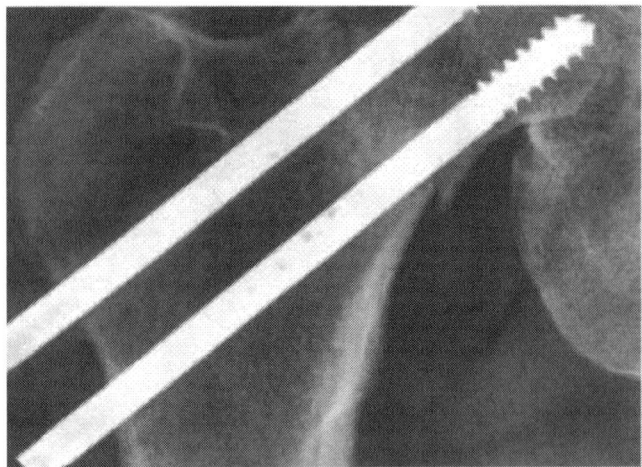

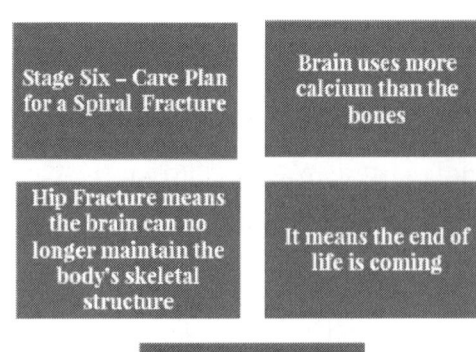

looking straight ahead. This ability is affected by dementia-caused damage in the occipital lobes. People who can't fully sense the environment around them are likely to trip, stumble, or fall over items dropped on the floor or clutter. They are likely to trip when trying to step onto a carpet or a rug. It's not uncommon to see a Person with Dementia backing up and bending to sit in a nonexistent chair because of damage in the occipital lobes.

A condition called occipital blindness may occur in some People with Dementia. In Stage Six of the disease, the right occipital lobe appears to turn off information from the left eye. That leaves the PWD with only a small tunnel of sight in the right eye. This vision change makes approaching the Person with Dementia from the front critical for all caregivers.

As research has progressed, much more has been learned about the way in which People with Dementia fall. In Alzheimer's, the person tends to attempt to rise out of a chair, lose her balance, but fall back into the chair. Obviously, these "falls" don't get recorded and are usually not even noticed by staff because there is no injury. Otherwise, she will fall when attempting to stand or walk because the brain can no longer provide the needed instruction to the body.

Brains with Vascular Damage

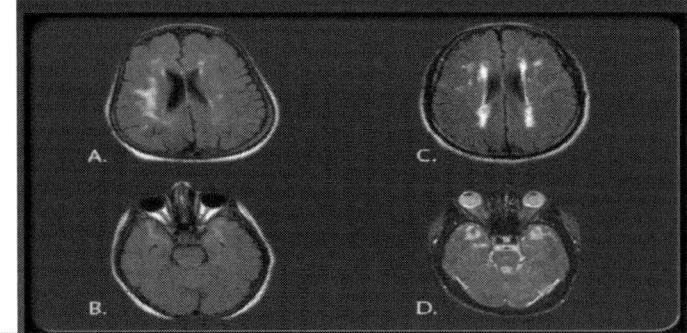

People with Vascular Dementias have a different experience when attempting to stand from a seated position. Vascular dementias frequently damage areas throughout the brain, causing even greater difficulty with movement. A person with Vascular Dementia may also lose her balance as she stands, but she has a higher risk of falling face forward out of the chair, rather than backwards. She continues the fall to the floor, landing on her face, elbows, and knees.

Because of the physiological response of the body to bruising, the facial bruise is particularly painful to see. In other areas of the body, bruises normally occur in areas with muscle cell structure. A bruise indicates a strike or insult to the body that resulted in a blood vessel rupturing or tearing, causing blood cells to spill into the muscle tissue. The abundance of cells in muscle tissue means the body is better able to respond to the damage. Over the course of several days, the dead blood cells are removed from the tissue and the bruise lightens, changes color, and finally disappears.

By contrast the face contains little musculature, leaving nowhere for the blood cells to absorb or hide in tissue. Instead, gravity pulls the dead blood cells down to the bottom of the face. Healing is much slower due to the lack of muscle tissue and blood vessels, though the dead blood cells are eventually removed. A blow or fall strike to the forehead easily turns into a slow, red, yellow, green, massive insult, then slowly moves down the face, finally disappearing at the jaw or neck.

People with Vascular Dementia are also prone to falls toward the weak side of the body when walking. Remember, the right side of the brain controls the left side of the body, and the left side of the brain controls the right side. While she is up and walking, anticipate she will fall toward the weaker side of her body, the side compromised by the stroke or vascular activity.

Lewy Bodies Dementias (LBD) or the Parkinson's Disease Dementias (PDD) also have unique falls related to where the brain damage has occurred. Unlike Alzheimer's and Vascular Dementias, these falls aren't related to sudden changes in blood pressure or motor damage, but to an area of the brain responsible for being awake and alert.

Lewy Bodies Dementias

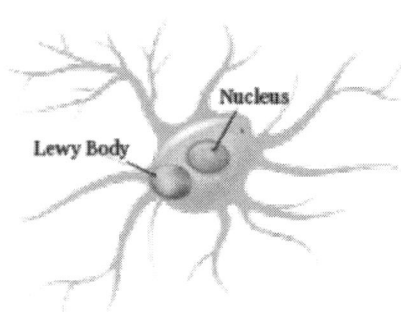

- Hallucinations (children, bugs, spiders, rats, snakes, bad guys coming to get me, spouse or caregiver having sex)
- REM sleep behavior disorder
- Systematized Delusions
- Sudden Intense Depression
- Fluctuating Cognition
- Deficits in attention & executive function
- Deficits in visuospatial function
- Repeated falls with head strikes
- Fainting (syncope)
- Unexplained loss of consciousness
- Very sensitive to medications
- Risk for sexual abuse of spouse if having sexual hallucinations

Persons with Lewy Bodies Dementias and Parkinson's Disease Dementias fall stiffly, like a board, standing up and suddenly falling forward, landing on their faces. If you witness this type of fall, it might surprise you to see that she doesn't put her hands out to catch herself. Likewise, while standing still, she will fall stiffly backwards, cracking the crown of her head, with no flailing of the arms as the fall occurs. Both unique falls happen because of where her brain is damaged. She falls because she suddenly loses consciousness, not because of a change in her blood pressure.

People with behavioral or communication FrontoTemporal Dementias (FTDs) may still be able to walk late in the disease but may walk in an awkward fashion. It is not unusual to see a person with FrontoTemporal Dementia bent forward from the waist while walking. This person is especially out of balance as the weight of the head, shoulders, and arms tip her headfirst into objects or onto the floor. She may have dozens of falls a day, with each fall possibly causing more damage to her brain due to ruptured vessels and bruising. She will also remove any headgear or helmets designed to protect her.

People with Wernicke-Korsakoff's Syndrome, the dementia most caused by alcohol abuse, may fall in any direction. It will depend on how long alcohol was abused and how damaged the brain has become.

People with Huntington's Disease or Huntington's Chorea may fall in any direction. For people with the limb-jerking motions of Huntington's, falls can be especially dangerous due to the force of the jerking limbs. So as the body falls, the thrashing movement of the limbs adds to the force of the fall.

People with Chronic Traumatic Encephalopathy (CTE) may have falls in any direction. Distinct forms of CTE are classified as Movement Forms, meaning

NOTES

Wernicke-Korsakoff's Syndrome

Wernicke
- Most will develop Wernicke's confusion
- Jerky eye movements
- Droopy upper eyelids
- Double vision
- Altered mental status
- Poor balance
- Difficulty walking
- May appear to be drunk when sober

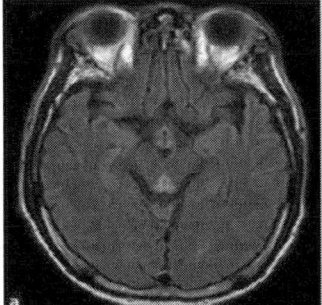
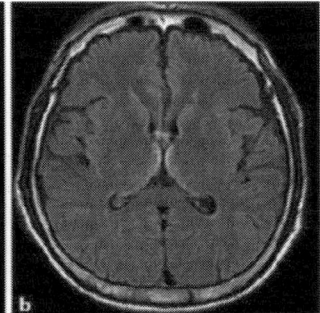

Korsakoff
- Memory loss
- Challenged to perform ALDs and IADLs
- Difficulty learning new information
- Confabulate information to fill in breaks/gaps in memory
- May be agitated and aggressive or withdrawn

Huntington's Dementia • Juvenile Huntington's • Huntington's Chorea

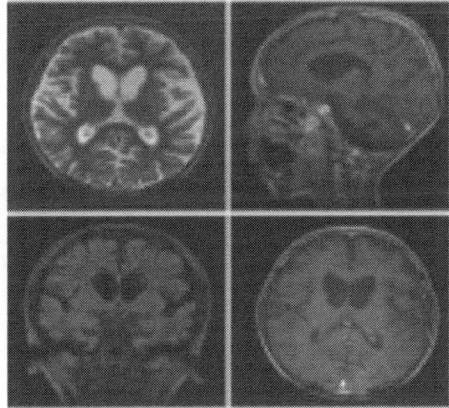
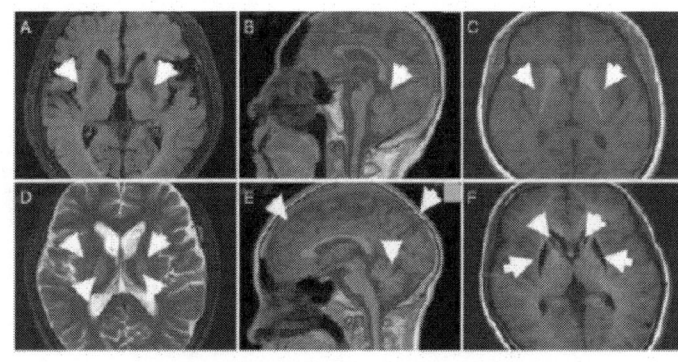

- Abnormal and jerking body movements (Chorea)
- Slow bodily movement
- Decreased muscle activity
- Fidgeting

- Declining cognitive skills
- Depression
- Irritability
- Anxiety
- Some may progress to exhibiting psychotic behaviors
- Inherited from parent

*CTE —
Chronic
Traumatic
Encephalopathy*

Young Onset
(Ages 18-35)
Late Onset
(Ages 60+)
- Movement
- Cognition
- Language
- Mood

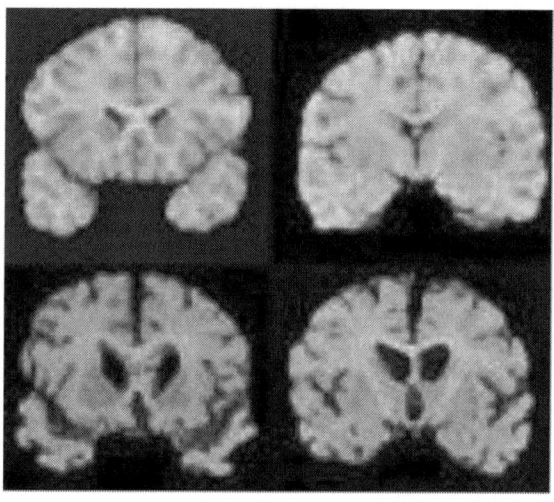

the areas of the brain responsible for coordinated and purposeful movement are especially damaged.

Everybody with dementia falls. It's a part of the disease, directly linked to brain damage. Some dementias cause falls to happen earlier in the disease process, some dementias are even partially identified by the person's type of fall. Some people will fall only a few times, while others will suffer daily impacts. It's another cruelty of a terrible disease.

Question 4: Has Your Loved One Had A Urinary Tract Infection (UTI) Yet?

Urinary tract infections (UTIs) are not only an ongoing scourge in dementia care, but they are also potentially deadly to the Person with Dementia. UTIs are greatly misunderstood by caregivers and medical professionals. Families, and even medical staff, often insist that UTIs are caused by the Person with Dementia having a soiled or wet brief. It's one of the most common myths I hear. The scenario is unpleasant, but it does exist in elder care. For People with Dementia, a soiled brief is not how the infection begins in the urinary tract. Rather, UTIs are directly linked to brain damage. UTIs are seen as a symptom of late-stage dementia.

People with Dementia begin to develop and continue to experience UTIs because of brain damage. By the end of the disease in Stage Seven, the UTIs may be detected, treated for 10 days, and the Person with Dementia will begin a new UTI within a few days.

As caregivers, knowing how many UTIs the Person with Dementia has had in the past two years is crucial. The third UTI occurring in a short time can indicate the presence of a super drug-resistant infection. The attending physician needs to know the frequency of UTIs to change the antibiotic with each new infection.

The causation of the UTIs is quite apparent, but often completely overlooked. The brain runs the body. As the brain suffers more damage, the body works less and less efficiently. You and I have a three-pound brain. We can fight infections, even infections you don't realize you have.

Our brain recognizes infection and begins a reaction in the body to destroy it. The brain alerts white blood cells and T cells to seek out, attack, and destroy the infection. The brain raises the body's core temperature to increase the effectiveness of the assault on the infection. As a result, we haven't been aware of the assault on our body's systems.

The Person with Dementia has a damaged brain. A damaged brain cannot run

---

Treatable Causes of Urinary Tract Incontinence — UTIs

D elirium

I nfection – urinary (symptomatic)

A tropic urethritis and vaginitis

P harmaceuticals

P sychologic disorders, especially depression

E xcessive urine output (eg, from heart failure or hyperglycemia)

R estricted mobility

S tool impaction

(Resnick, NM: "Urinary incontinence in the elderly." Medical Grand Rounds 3:281-290, 1984.)

the body effectively. A damaged brain is less and less capable of telling the body how to function.

As the disease of dementia progresses, the body temperature in a Person with Dementia also begins to fall. The damage in the parietal lobes makes it hard to raise the core temperature to the normal temperature of 98.6 degrees. In Stage Five of the disease, the Person with Dementia will begin to have a lower body temperature, usually between 97 and 95 degrees. Death occurs at 93 degrees, so a Person with Dementia would be in Stage Seven and near the end of life with a temperature of 95.

As less and less healthy brain tissue remains, a correlating drop in the brain's ability to respond and protect the body occurs. Infections experienced by People with Dementia are especially concerning due to the brain's inability to respond. UTIs quickly overwhelm the body's systems, leading to sepsis (blood overwhelmed by infection), and the sepsis leads to kidney failure (renal failure), which leads to death. Sepsis is commonly called "blood poisoning" because infection poisons the blood beyond the body's ability to remove it.

Caregivers who are alert to sudden changes in their loved one's behavior should immediately notify the physician and, using the hat method (a plastic cup that fits on the toilet bowl to catch urine), attempt to collect a urine sample when the Person with Dementia toilets. Hospitalization may be needed in some People with Dementia, depending to how much healthy brain tissue can respond to each new infection.

Some research theorizes the Person with Dementia is unable to effectively destroy the infection, in spite of the antibiotics. This would create the possibility

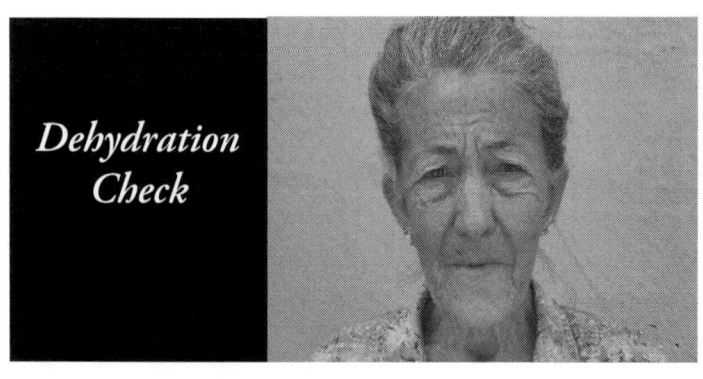

Dehydration Check

- Can't pinch skin?
- Its too loose and no longer snappy?
- Press your thumb firmly between her eyes, just above the eyebrows.
- Count to five and quickly move your thumb.
- It there is a white area where your thumb was, she needs fluids!

that the Person with Dementia is carrying a low-grade infection that can suddenly overwhelm the body's ability to fight it.

Communities, especially memory care communities, train caregivers to be alert to the signs of infection and UTIs. Operating under a medical model, People with Dementia are encouraged to drink fluids at all mealtimes. Additional hydration stations or carts are utilized in between meals to continue to encourage water intake.

Fluids are offered during activities, following exercise, and at bedtime. However, urinary tract infections for People with Dementia are usually not related to the fluid intake; they are related to brain damage and the brain's resulting inability to produce a normal immune response.

Question 5: How Guilty do You Feel?

One of the most stressful decisions family caregivers faces involves placement of a loved one in a care facility. Several factors are at work in these situations.

Typically, care has been provided for a decade or more, and the family caregiver is physically and emotionally exhausted. The caregiver may worry about the opinions of others, paying for care, or believe their loved one's behaviors may be too challenging. Spouses and relatives may see placement as the breaking of wedding vows.

Cultural issues for African American, Hispanic American, Asian American, and other families may mean facing severe backlash for placing a loved one under professional care. Members of the family, church members, neighbors, and other friends may view the move as abandonment rather than an attempt to get a loved one the specialized medical care they need.

Addressing guilt — the elephant in the room — is critical for developing a successful partnership of care. Many people have promised loved ones that they will never place them in a nursing home, having made this promise without realizing that a dementia diagnosis eventually requires specialized, around-the-clock medical care.

By Stage Five, People with Dementia require a great deal of reminders, hands-on assistance, socialization, exercise, care, and patience. In Stage Six, two caregivers may be required for transfers, bathing, and toileting. Stage Seven means two or more caregivers may be required to provide full-time care for the Person with Dementia. This level of intense care is physically challenging and mentally and emotionally exhausting as well.

Families may also face the pressure of social expectations that demand caring for a loved one at home. African Americans and Hispanic Americans have the highest risks for Vascular Dementias and the least support for care. As they explore external care resources, they may see a loss in social standing or family backlash. Some experience shaming from friends and relatives, from places of worship, or from their neighbors — all for seeking the facility care that a loved one may desperately need.

It is important to support families in their decision to seek care of a loved one from medical professionals. We should encourage them to join support groups and praise them for their loyalty and concern for a loved one.

People who shame caregivers about seeking outside assistance show a lack of education about the disease, a lack of awareness of its impact on the Person with Dementia, and a lack of understanding about the physical, mental, and emotional impacts on caregivers. The stress caregivers face is dangerous. A 2020 study by the AARP found an estimated three in 10 family caregivers die

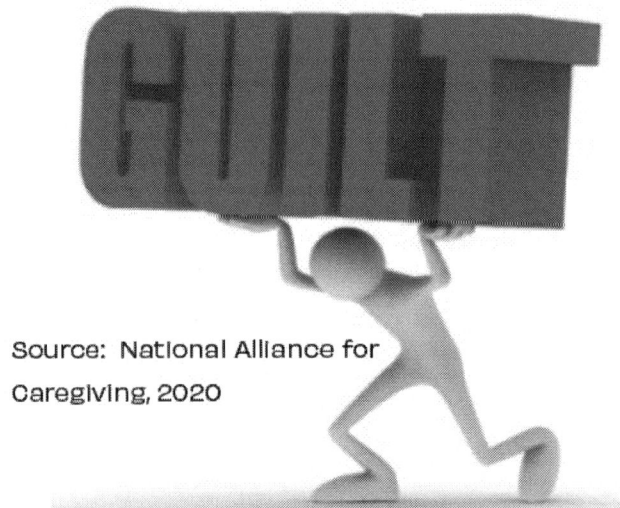

30% of family caregivers die before the person they are caring for.

Source: National Alliance for Caregiving, 2020

before their loved ones, due to the stress of care.

However, once a Person with Dementia needs placement with professional caregivers, will the family come back for breakfast, lunch, or dinner? Will they visit on holidays, birthdays, parties, and education nights? Will this family continue to visit and treat the Person with Dementia as an honored family member?

If the answers are "yes," then the family and the caregiver need to let the guilt go. No one in the family expected dementia. No one knew it would happen, and no one understands what the family caregiver faces, except for other family caregivers and perhaps the professional caregiver.

The move into a community should allow the family caregiver to return to being a spouse, a son, or a daughter. Time together can be spent sharing a slice of pie or watching an old movie, not changing an underwear brief, or arguing about a dirty shirt.

Don't discount the level of stress suffered by the family caregiver. That crabby, short-tempered, exhausted person may be providing dementia care, working a full-time job, and providing for children at home. The caregiver suffers from significant stress that can cause an increased risk of death. Honesty and openness about the care the Person with Dementia needs gives families the blessing they require to seek professional care.

Support Groups

Investigating professional care facilities is a challenging and emotional process. Feelings of guilt are common, and caregivers may or may not receive the support of families and communities throughout this difficult process. Support groups can provide a positive counter experience by providing information, referrals, and lessons from experience that can offset the negative feedback from others. The family caregiver's health is at risk during this disease, and a support group can often save the caregiver's life.

Five Things to Remember

1. The brain runs the body. As the brain becomes more and more damaged, the body works less effectively.

2. Most falls are likely to happen because of brain damage to the motor cortex, premotor cortex and the limbic system. Other falls are related to the sudden loss of consciousness.

3. Urinary tract infections (UTIs) are caused by damage to the brain. When UTIs become chronic, it indicates the brain has become too damaged to monitor and fight infection.

4. Each lobe of the brain has certain duties, and when that lobe becomes damaged, the Person with Dementia will display different behaviors.

5. When a Person with Dementia begins to have difficulty chewing and swallowing food, the disease is now in the brain stem.

NOTES

$\mathcal{T}wo$
THE LOBES OF THE BRAIN

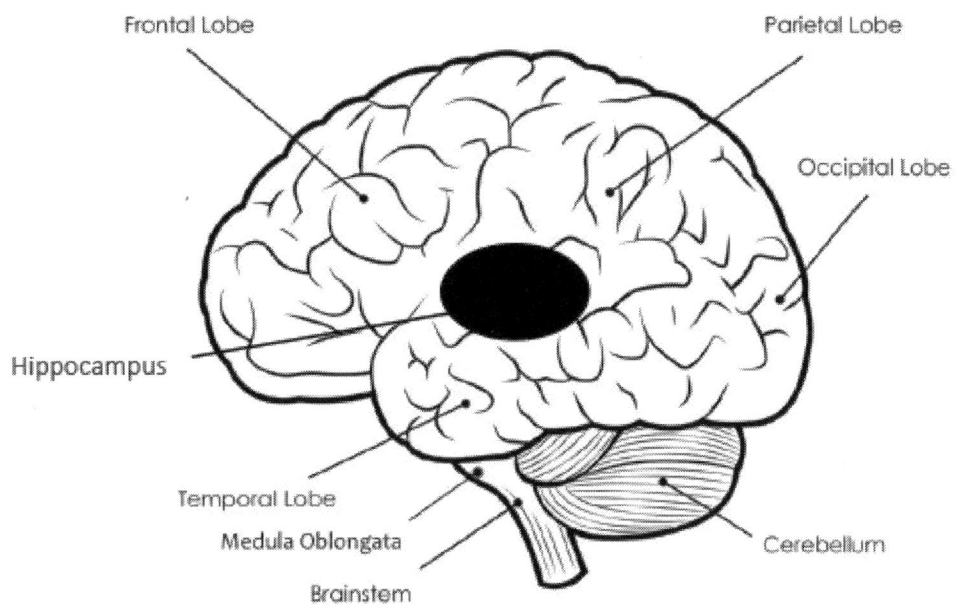

The brain contains seven sets of lobes and weighs about three pounds. The brain runs the body and contains the personality that makes you who you are. The brain produces chemicals used by the brain and the body — electrical impulses firing within the cell structures, white matter, gray matter, neurons, proteins, and pathways connecting the different lobes to each other.

The lobes of the brain contain a matched set, or identical lobes on each side of the brain. The left side lobes control the right side of the body. The right lobes control the left side of the body. Generally, both sides perform similar actions, although some lobes appear to have different functions.

Understanding what each lobe is responsible for helps us understand how the lobes affect a person's normal function. We can begin to recognize how behaviors in People with Dementia will change as each lobe suffers damage. Knowledge of the brain's functions allows us to determine where brain damage is occurring and why changes are occurring.

Hippocampus and Limbic System

Memories begin in the hippocampus and limbic system of the brain. When these areas function incorrectly, a person cannot learn or retain new information. If a person appears cold to a new grandchild, it doesn't mean she does not love her new great grandchild. It means she is missing a piece of her brain that makes memory of that child work.

To make matters worse, her coldness toward the child may typically occur when she does not appear physically ill. She won't appear that way until Stage Six of the disease. It's common for family caregivers to believe she is behaving in a bothersome manner and is trying to be purposefully annoying.

Once the hippocampus becomes damaged, the Person with Dementia will likely ask the same questions or repeat behavior again and again without realizing she is doing so.

No matter how many times you repeat the information, she will not be able to learn or retain it. The area of her brain that makes memory no longer functions, and the ability to remember information will eventually go away entirely.

Which of the A's of Dementia do you see when the Hippocampus is damaged?
Amnesia

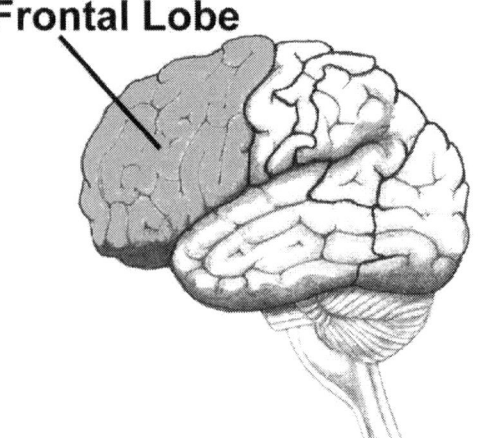

Amnesia is the inability to use or retain memory, including short-term and long-term memory. The person may constantly repeat questions such as "Where am I?" and "Who are you?" or "When are we going to eat?" She may accuse the caregiver of stealing or being an impostor. This type of behavior can continue for hours at a time and occurs due to damage in the frontal lobes and the hippocampus.

The Frontal Lobe System

The frontal lobes store memory, personality, cognition, impulse control, speech, attention, rational thought, imagination, and judgment. The hippocampus allows us to learn new information, such as being able to answer the question "Where are we going?"

Amnesia is usually the first area of change noticed by families and the "A" which has most likely caused verbal or physical abuse within the family structure. As amnesia begins, the Person with Dementia does not look ill, so her confusion and inability to remember things can appear purposeful. The Person with Dementia's behaviors are often interpreted as just "annoying," rather than a warning sign of the disease and its progression in the brain.

Normal Function of the Frontal Lobe includes abstract thought, personality, attention, behavior, sexual behavior, emotional expression, initiation, concentration, organization, motor planning, self-monitoring, awareness of ability, coordination of movement, creative thought, imagination, impulse control, inhibition, initiative, intellect, judgment, memory, problem solving, the ability to produce and understand language, rational thought, reflection, speech, and some emotion.

Symptoms of Frontal Lobe Impairment:
- Changes in personality & social behavior
- Loss of spontaneity in interactions
- Loss of flexibility in thinking
- Sequencing – inability to complete tasks in the right order
- Easily distracted
- Mood swings
- Diminished abstract reasoning
- Difficulty with problem solving
- Language difficulties – word usage and word finding
- Loss of simple movement in various parts of the body
- Perseveration – repeating actions or comments without awareness

Which of the A's of the Dementia do you usually see when the Frontal Lobe is damaged?

Anger, apathy, attention, anxiety — these are often witnessed as the Person with Dementia begins to react to her brain's failure to function normally. Anxiety and anger may come in short outbursts with no recall of the behavior. Frustrated by the brain's failure to secure needed information, a typical reaction is agitated behavior, with no recognition of brain failure. Pointing out this inability to produce the correct thought or action typically results in the Person with Dementia becoming annoyed with the caregiver. You may feel her anger full force if you insist on pointing out the deficits in her thinking. Since she is not aware that her thought processes are incorrect, she will naturally believe you are trying to trick or fool her.

Temporal Lobe System

The temporal lobes control hearing, language, and sense of smell. The left lobe is believed to control formal language and the right lobe to control automatic speech (yes and no), singing, and forbidden or hateful words, including cursing. The left lobe is generally destroyed first, leaving the Person with Dementia only the ability to communicate with swearing and singing.

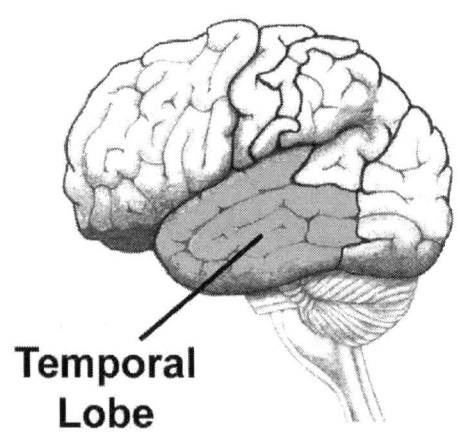

Normal Function of the Temporal Lobe includes auditory memories, cursing, fear, hearing, understanding, language, music, awareness, sense of identity, singing, some behavior and emotion, feelings, organization and sequencing, sense of smell, some visual pathways, speech, and visual memories (faces, places, foods, objects), memory, learning, and information retrieval.

Symptoms of Temporal Lobe Impairment:
- Difficulty remembering names and faces
- Difficulty with identification and verbalization of objects
- Difficulty understanding the spoken word
- Concentration difficulties
- Aggressive behavior
- Short-term memory loss
- Long-term memory loss
- Change in sexual interest
- Persistent talking
- Difficulty locating objects in the environment
- Inability to categorize objects
- Religiosity
- Seizure disorders, auras, and strange reveries

Which of the A's of the Dementia do you usually see when the Temporal Lobe is damaged?

Aphasia

The inability to use or understand language is called aphasia. The person will use the wrong word, or complete a story with phrases from another story, or provide a lengthy description of an item because she cannot find the right word. She may call family members by the wrong name, which increases the family's anxiety and concern. This word-finding difficulty will increase until all language ability is lost. This is associated with damage to the temporal lobes and the frontal lobes.

Occipital Lobe System

The occipital lobes are responsible for translating the visual imagery sent from the eye. These two lobes translate the information from each eye into a three-dimensional image and connect that image to the appropriate memory. Eyeglasses are not part of the visual translation. Rather, they function to force a muscle in the eye to constrict causing the signal to be in focus for the occipital lobes. Vision loss is not due to a poor eyeglass prescription, but to progressive damage to the brain.

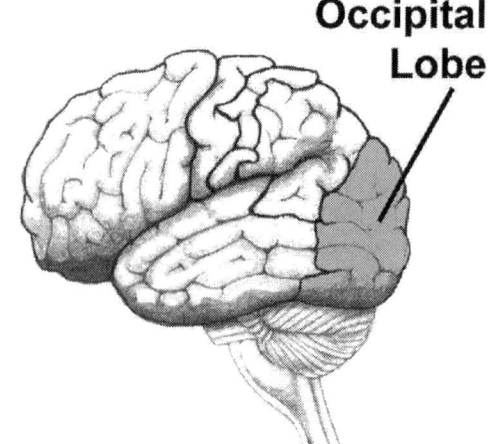

Occipital Lobe

Normal occipital lobe function includes depth perception, facial recognition, visual reception area, reading, visual acuity, and visual interpretation.

Symptoms of Occipital Lobe Impairment:
- Impaired vision
- Front visual fields impacted
- Progression of 3D to 1D
- Possible loss of vision in left eye
- Peripheral vision field is reduced
- Misinterpretation of persons, objects, and environment

Which of the A's of the Dementia do you usually see when the Occipital Lobe is damaged?

Agnosia

The inability to recognize people or use common objects is called agnosia. The person may become lost in a familiar place because she doesn't recognize the items that alert her to the surroundings. She may confuse a fork with a spoon, a toothbrush with a hairbrush, or toothpaste with denture cream. Eventually, she loses the ability to recognize objects completely.

The person may also confuse memories of a son with a husband or a father or an uncle. She may confuse her daughter with a mother or an aunt or a grandmother. This process is associated with increased damage to the frontal lobes, the occipital lobes (visual association, distance, and depth perception) and the temporal lobes. Memory is lost in a reverse order of being learned. A Person with Dementia may think she is 40 even though she is 80.

If her memories only go back to age 40, she will attempt to identify family members by assigning them the identity of the family member who most closely meets their expected appearance and age. In other words, great grandchildren may be confused with her children because the ages of the great grandchildren match her current age-40 memories.

The process of dementia reverses the order of learning in most people. Maslow and Eriksen's scales of development go from infancy to adulthood. The Alzheimer's Retro-Genesis Scale (*retro* – back to and *genesis* – the beginning) means the Person with Dementia will slowly lose memories from adulthood back to infancy. Old memory or long-term memory or lifetime memory, the building blocks of our files of knowledge, become our last memories. Basically, a Person with Dementia may know where she was raised, but not where she is in the present time.

Parietal Lobe

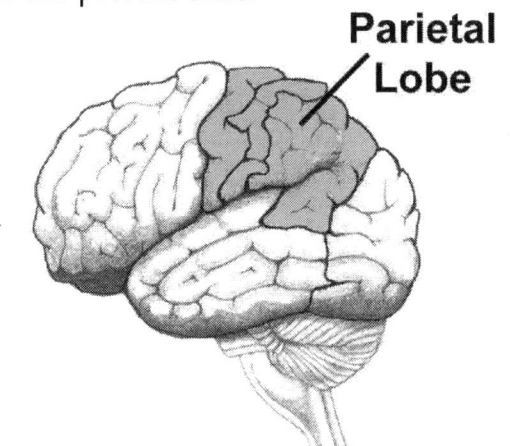

The parietal lobes control pain, touch, taste, and body temperature. Recognizing infection and responding with an increase in the body's core temperature is controlled and monitored here. As the disease progresses, damage to this lobe will cause the Person with Dementia to have a much lower body temperature.

Normal function of the parietal lobe includes monitoring the body's temperature perception, sensory combination, and comprehension. Normal function also includes writing and reading, some visual functions, taste and touch, math calculations, academic skills, visual perception, spatial perception, differentiation of shape, size, and color, and sense of touch, taste, smell.

Symptoms of Parietal Lobe Impairment:
- Difficulty naming objects
- Difficulty writing words
- Difficulty multitasking
- Problems with reading
- Poor hand-eye coordination

- Confusion with left-right orientation
- Difficulty with math and drawing
- Poor visual perception – the inability to focus visual attention
- Lack of awareness of body and space
- Lower body temperature
- The person may be left with only the ability to taste sweets and frequently begins to crave sweets because it's all she can taste.

Which of the A's of the Dementia do you usually see when the Parietal Lobe is damaged?

Apraxia

The inability to use or coordinate purposeful muscle movement is called apraxia. In the early stages, the person may reach for an item and miss it. She may have difficulty catching a ball or clapping her hands. The floor may appear to be moving to this person and balance becomes affected, increasing the risk for falls and injury. In time, this loss of ability to move affects the Activities of Daily Living (transferring, sleeping, walking, toileting, bathing, grooming, dressing, and eating). In the end stage, the person is not able to properly chew or swallow food, increasing the risk of choking or aspiration. This is linked to damage to parietal lobes (pain, touch, temperature and pressure, sensory perception), the cortex (skilled movement), and the occipital lobes.

Cerebellum and Medulla Oblongata Systems

These minor lobes help with coordination and control of coordinated movements, balance and muscle tone, equilibrium, and some memory of reflex motor acts.

Symptoms of Cerebellum and Medulla Oblongata Impairment:
- Tremors
- Involuntary eye movements
- Ataxia – the lack of coordination
- Weak muscles
- Inability to judge distance and when to stop

- Inability to perform rapid altering movement
- Slurred speech

Normal medulla oblongata functions help regulate breathing, heart and blood vessel function, digestion, sneezing, swallowing, respiration, and circulation.

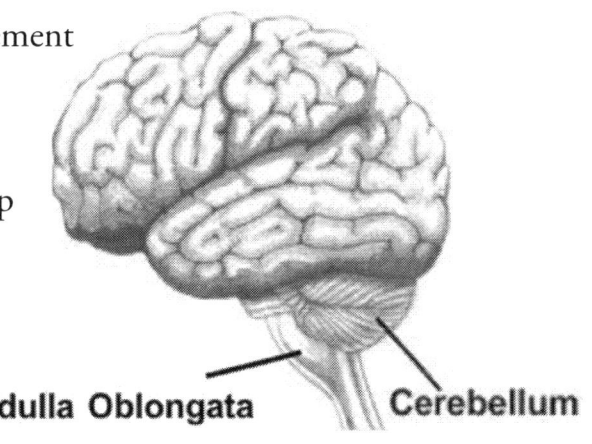

Symptoms of Medulla Oblongata Impairment:
- Communication between the brain and the spinal cord is disrupted.
- In chronic alcohol use, significant synapse loss and axonal impairment makes the brain susceptible to injury.
- Swallowing food and liquids.
- Swallowing plays a role in heart rate, reflexes to sight and sound, sweating, blood pressure, digestion, temperature, levels of alertness, ability to sleep, and balance.

Brain Stem System

Brain Stem Symptoms of Impairment:
- Difficulty swallowing food and liquids
- Dizziness and nausea
- Sleeping difficulties
- Decreased breathing capacity
- Problems with balance and movement
- Difficulty with organization and/or perception of the environment

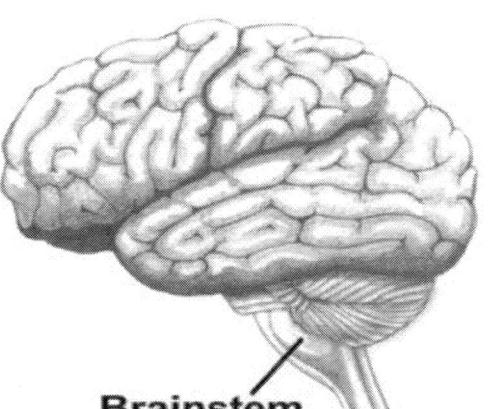

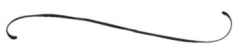

FIVE THINGS TO REMEMBER   NOTES

1. The brain controls the body.

2. Each lobe of the brain is responsible for certain behaviors, actions, movements, and more.

3. When these areas are damaged, we can tell which lobe is impacted by the behaviors displayed by the Person with Dementia.

4. Persons with Dementia are not aware their brain is damaged.

5. Persons with Dementia are simply responding to their brain.

Three
WHAT IS MEMORY?

Memory is a complex process of how the brain's systems respond to stimuli and encoding the information into different lobes, neurons, and other cellular structures or areas of the brain. Some functional areas of the brain are still not fully understood. Connections between systems remain unidentified; yet they are critical to understanding and resolving the damage done by dementia. To help, we will review some brain physiology, aging theory, family dynamics, and educational psychology.

I'll start by breaking memory into what people think it means. Next, you'll learn about the three types of memory, before moving into an exploration of neurons and other aspects of the brain including, how memory is made, and finally, how memory gets destroyed. We will bring it all together in The File Cabinet Analogy to help you fully understand what is happening to your loved one's memory.

What People Think Memory Means

In the diagnosis process, many families have been told that the course of dementia will cause their loved one to lose their memory. Most families think this memory loss will mean forgetfulness, possibly an inability to follow a conversation or learn a new grandchild's name. They may believe memory loss means the loved one will become unsafe to drive a car. These things certainly happen to the Person with Dementia.

The family receives little information on what "memory" really means or how the disease will progress. Families are generally not aware how the ability to retrieve, recall, and store or encode information affects behaviors. For memory to work and for new memory to be encoded, the brain must be whole and intact with a functioning hippocampus and limbic system. Dementias destroy these areas of the brain. Dementias cause massive cellular and system damage globally, meaning the damage from dementia is eventually found throughout the brain.

Persons with Dementia who survive to Stage 7 of the disease (referred to medically as Very Severe Dementia) will have lost almost two pounds of an original three-pound brain. The loss of brain structures and systems includes the hippocampus and limbic systems.

Consequently, the Person with Dementia may at times exhibit challenging behaviors, such as "refusing" to bathe or to stop driving a car. Families may be fooled about the loved one's true abilities because People with Dementia don't look physically ill until Stage 6 of the disease (Severe Dementia). Family members may believe that their loved one understands how to drive or take a bath but is "choosing" to be difficult.

Caregivers can believe the Person with Dementia is "pretending" memory loss in interactions with the doctor or to others. This happens because the loved one relies on brain "files" containing social skills that were created in childhood. The doctor politely asks, "How are you?" of the Person with Dementia. This triggers the long-term memory of a long-ingrained greeting. It's not a true conversation, just the repetition of learned conversation by responding, "Fine."

The lack of education and understanding about dementia can have dire consequences. I have been repeatedly told by angry families that their loved one is pretending or "showing off" for the doctor when the person was simply responding with a long-term memory and social skill.

Memory loss affects other areas of life as well. A wife told me recently that her husband could still "basically" drive, but since he appeared to have "lost his nerve," she was forcing him to continue to attempt to drive. It was a "man up" approach, I suppose, but ultimately dangerous for him and her and other travelers.

He hadn't lost his confidence about driving. He was afraid because a part of him recognized that other cars move too fast, and there are too many stimuli for his brain to assess and respond effectively. He felt afraid and scared about being in a car as a passenger, much less being the driver.

Families also mistakenly believe their loved one "knows" not to leave the neighborhood. These misconceptions arise from a lack of understanding of how dementia-induced brain damage affects a person's behaviors. It can lead to terrible outcomes.

A lady who "knows" how to drive to church and back home ends up several states away. In truth, she now operates with significant brain damage. You can't see the damage, of course, except in the person's behaviors.

Families believe the Person with Dementia can "remember" to take medications but is purposefully electing not to do so. Again, this is untrue. The damage to the brain prevents a Person with Dementia from remembering what, when and how.

People with Dementia suffer from falls because of brain damage, specifically the destruction of the limbic system, premotor cortex, and motor cortex. They aren't pretending to move awkwardly to be difficult, they fall because these areas of the brain are too damaged to function or no longer exist.

Once enough of the lobes are damaged, Persons with Dementia may become confrontational, annoyed, or verbally or physically challenging. They may display a change in personality. Brain damage is the true causation of the behaviors or the response to a caregiver. The Person with Dementia is doing the best she can with significant brain damage. Caregivers who accept this fact can begin to improve their techniques for providing care.

None of the behavior displayed by a Person with Dementia is purposeful. It doesn't matter what the behavior is, it is rooted in brain damage. It's that simple.

People do believe and often insist that a particular behavior is intentional or purposeful. I often tell families that if they explain to a stranger, or a family member, or a medical professional, that their loved one has brain cancer, they will get understanding, kindness, and support. Tell those same people the disease is dementia and prepare for the opposite to happen. It's because people don't understand the Person with Dementia is losing brain tissue.

Memory means the ability to walk, to move the body, to understand how to complete the Activities of Daily Living or ADLs. The ADLs measure a person's ability to transfer themselves from a lying position, to sitting, to a standing position, to ambulate or walk, to toilet, to bathe, to groom, to dress, and to eat.

Families don't realize that their loved one will lose the ability to do the Instrumental Activities of Daily Living or IADLs. These include being able to use a phone, shop, prepare food, perform normal housekeeping, do laundry, use public transportation or drive a car, take medications correctly, and handle finances.

Mishandled finances are particularly dangerous. I've known families who lost millions of dollars because no one was watching, or the adult children didn't feel comfortable stepping in and taking over. I know of families who lost everything they had saved because no one was aware the Person with Dementia was using the computer during the day and was giving money away. This occurs because no one recognized or understood that People with Dementia do not look physically sick until the end of the disease, yet the brain is heavily damaged.

Financial control cannot safely remain in the hands of the Person with Dementia. Houses get refinanced, accounts are emptied, strangers take money, or they fall victim to unscrupulous friends or family. Mail scams, telephone scams, or social media scams are not uncommon.

Some financial behaviors can seem harmless at first. Family caregivers may also be too physically and mentally drained to recognize the danger.

A wife called me recently. She was overwhelmed by the care she was providing to her parents and husband, all with different forms of dementia, and was physically and mentally exhausted. She had all the symptoms of compassion fatigue.

As she prepared to hang up, she remembered to ask me about her husband's recent behavior. He had been spending large amounts of money on new cars. Yet he would quickly — sometimes within hours — decide he didn't like the car and would trade it in for another. He had bought and traded several cars over a five-month period, each time complaining about a feature he couldn't understand like the stereo, self-parking, navigation screen and camera, locks, and the push-button starter.

The wife was extremely exhausted by her care giving duties, and didn't realize, until our conversation, that her husband was operating with a brain disease, and it was burning up their savings. She had argued endlessly with him that his car swapping made no sense. Not once did she connect this new and bizarre behavior to brain damage.

Families and professionals don't realize memory is not only who you are as a person, but it is also the ability to recall family members, stories about your life, or the thousands of tiny steps required for full functioning in daily life.

At the end of the disease, the loss of memory includes the inability to fight off infection and so urinary tract infections, or UTIs, become a danger.

Finally, the loss of memory will affect the very primitive brain stem, and the ability to properly chew and swallow food will be lost. Death from dementia is often caused by food particles being aspirated into the lungs, leading to aspiration pneumonia. This type of lung infection causes the blood to become septic or poisonous, which in turn leads to renal or kidney failure and death.

Three Forms of Memory

There are three types of memory in humans: **Long-Term Memory (LTM)**, **Short-Term Memory (STM)**, and **Sensory Memory (SM)**. Let's review what is known.

The process of receiving, securing, encoding, storing, and retrieving the impressions, experiences, and pieces of what we have studied or accumulated during our lives is called memory. We all share these forms of memory.

Long-term memory (LTM), also called lifetime memory, consists of all the memories stored up over an entire life. These memories provide a foundation for many abilities, including the Activities of Daily Living (ADLs), social skills, family recognition, life history, education, driving, reading, short-term memory (STM), and sensory memory. Long-term memory contains other more specific forms or types of memory.

As the fetal brain forms, as many as 200 billion neuron cells are created, but half are discarded as the fetus matures to birth. The best cells remain, leaving humans with approximately 100 billion neuron cells.

One part of the brain is referred to as the primal brain, sometimes called the primitive brain or the reptilian brain. It is responsible for survival, drive, and instinctual behaviors. The primal brain includes the brain stem, basal ganglia, the limbic system (amygdala, thalamus, corpus callosum, olfactory bulb, septum, entorhinal cortex, hippocampus, hypothalamus, and the fornix).

The information around us enters the brain through the sensory systems of vision, touch, hearing, smell, and taste. Let's use the example of a newborn coming into your family.

For months, information about the pregnancy has been coming into your hippocampus and limbic systems. News about the pregnancy, updates from doctor's visits, a grainy photo of a gray head and face in utero, the sex of the baby, the due date, baby showers, etc. Each bit of news or update about the baby formed a memory and added to the growth of dendrites on the brain's neurons. (Neurons will be explained next.)

The stimuli of each of these activities of information are translated into neurotransmitters, or chemicals, by the brain's neurons and fired electrically to the hippocampus and limbic systems, which determine the value of the information. The value determines whether it will be treated as long-term memory or short-term memory or sensory memory?

After determining whether this information is something needed for a few seconds or longer, or whether it is sensory information and requires immediate action ("Oh that's hot! Ouch!), it is either discarded or sent via more neurotransmitters through the brain's structures. The information travels to the desired lobe of the brain where similar information is located, and to the final neurons which will receive and encode or store the memory.

Sensory Memory is a mental representation of how the environment looks, feels, sounds, smells, and tastes. This includes auditory or **echoic memory, haptic**

NOTES

memory, or **touch memory** (how the fur of your dog feels), and visual or **iconic memory**. (Smell and taste memory are not as well studied.) Short-term memory is the working memory of the environment around you and lasts between 30 seconds to one minute before the hippocampus discards the stimuli. It stores your interpretation of the event.

Long-Term Memory is comprised of additional forms of memory, divided into explicit memory or implicit memory. Other types of memory systems stem from these two categories.

Explicit Memory (also called conscious memory) are memories formed by the hippocampus and medial temporal lobe systems. These are memories you must consciously work to recall, they are not automatic memories. Explicit memory is further subdivided into declarative memory, a memory of facts, events, things you learned in school, etc. Memory of emotional events are stored here, but the expression of the emotion is retrieved from implicit memory.

Declarative Memory is further split into either episodic memory or semantic memory. **Episodic memory** holds the events and experiences you recall about your life. This includes memories of your birthday, how you learned about the attacks of 9/11 and the World Trade Centers, what you ate for lunch yesterday, the party you enjoyed with your best friend.

Semantic Memory includes facts and concepts, knowledge about the world, vocabulary, numbers, and general knowledge intertwined with experiences. You don't recall learning most of your semantic memory.

Implicit Memory is memory you don't have to think about. It is the automatic response to events. It affects thoughts and behaviors. This memory is further defined as **procedural memory**. This is the part of memory that allows you to do everyday things without thinking about them.

Procedural Memory is heavily damaged in dementia. The memory that allows you to perform the Activities of Daily Living enables you to do routine tasks without thinking. When a Person with Dementia begins to fail on the dozens of steps required to transfer, ambulate, toilet, bath, groom, dress, and eat, our

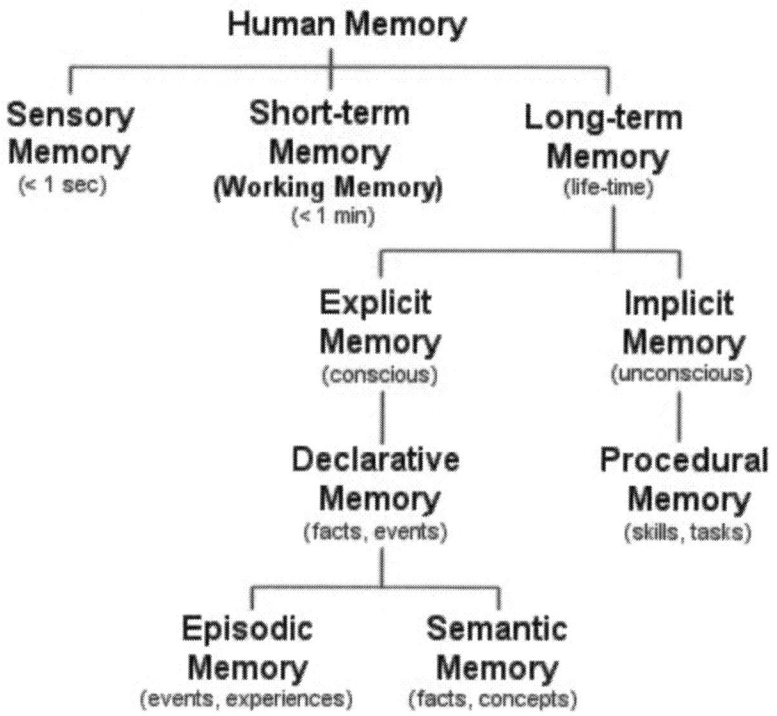

common response is to believe the person is doing the behavior on purpose to be annoying.

Again, brain damage causes these automatic tasks to become lost. To take a bath, you must first realize you need a bath. Bathing itself requires more than four dozen steps. The instructions for bathing also include being able to find the bathroom, being able to undress (belts, bras, socks, zippers, buttons, pullovers, underwear, etc.), turning on water to the right temperature, plugging the bathtub, and later draining water from the bathtub. The Person with Dementia must remember how to use soap, shampoo, conditioner, washcloth, and then properly rinse the body and hair, etc.

After the bath, the Person with Dementia must remember all the steps for how to dress again. For example, it takes three more steps to put a bra back on than it did to take it off! Bathing is our most complex Activity of Daily Living!

When procedural memory works, you and I are unaware of the complexity of the ADLs. Think about riding a bike, driving a car, taking a bath, making a meal, locking the doors, staying safe during bad weather, and all the other things we do without realizing our brain function allows these things to happen. Then imagine how different the world is when we can no longer automatically do these things.

As the disease progresses, our procedural memory has wasted away, requiring the dementia caregiver to provide much more assistance, and at the end of life, total care for the Person with Dementia.

Neurons and Other Stuff in the Brain

Neurons are the longest living cells in the body. As we age and continue to stay active, the dendrites on neurons continue to grow. By the time we reach mature adulthood in our 30s, some of our neurons now have dendrites several inches long.

Weighing three pounds, the brain is comprised of dozens of types of proteins, neurotransmitters, or chemicals produced by neurons, and other brain structures. There are an estimated 100 billion neuron or nerve cells and 360 billion additional cells called non-neural glial cells. These cells perform trillions of activities per nanosecond, a complex and vibrant pulsing action that keeps us moving and thinking accurately.

Neurotransmitters are part of the chemicals of the brain that allow the neurons to function and the brain to work.

Three Types of Neurons

Sensory Neurons receive information from the five senses.
Interneuron Cells bring information back and forth between the brain and spinal cord.
Motor Neurons send information to the muscle structure of the body.

The complexity of the brain and its parts can be difficult to grasp. Each of the 100 billion neurons is made up of hundreds or thousands of components. Each tiny piece is critical to the proper and correct function of the cell, thus the system, thus the brain, thus the memory, thus the body's function.

If key proteins in and around the neuron fail, the neuron malfunctions and ultimately dies. In the beginning stage of dementia, the brain has many fully functioning neurons, and families may not notice any changes in their loved one's

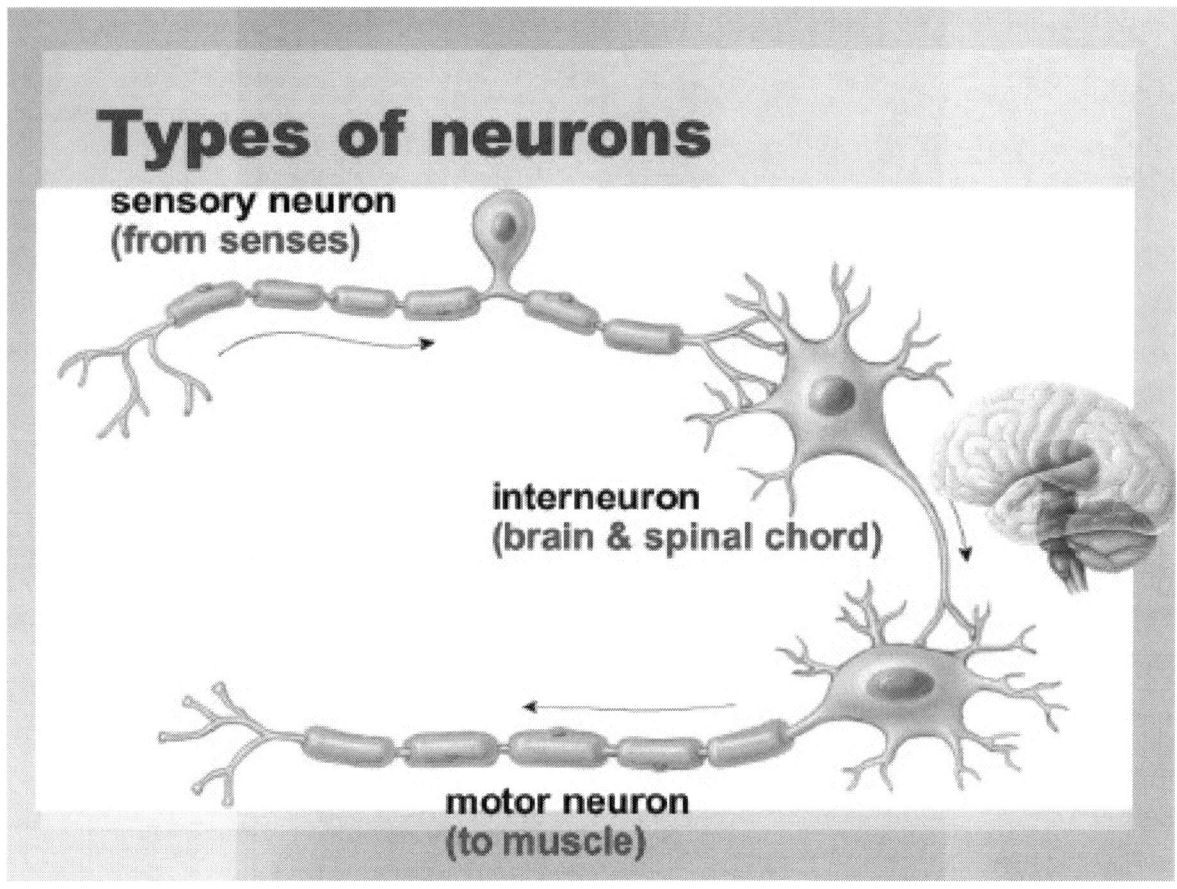

behavior.

As additional damage occurs; the loss of bits and pieces of cell parts and structures means memories begin to fail. Parts of one story get mixed with other stories. Dementias never stop progressing. Increasing parts of memory or ability become damaged and destroyed. Finally, the entire memory system is lost as cells continue to die. (When neurons die, they are removed from the body in waste.)

Our neurons are not simple-cell organisms. They are complex, comprised of thousands of pieces, and are parts of even more microscopic structures.

The illustration (*next page*) is a basic neuron magnified approximately 20,000 times above it's normal size. To put that into context, if a single piece of human hair was magnified 20,000 times, the hair would be six feet wide.

To view the structures that make up the neuron requires a much higher magnification. The level needed to see these tiny bits and pieces requires 100,000 times the magnification. That same strand of hair would then be 30 feet wide by comparison. (*next page*)

Neurons are the information messengers in the brain. By using the electrical charges of the brain, they produce or move chemicals to transfer signals carrying information between the different structures or systems of the brain, or between the brain and the rest of the nervous system, or to the muscles.

Everything we think and feel is because of the activity of our neurons and the two forms of glial cells, the microglia, astrocytes, and the oligodendrocytes. Each of these various forms of cells surround and support the healthy function of the three forms of neurons we rely on. Glial cells work in conjunction with blood vessel cells to regulate brain function and support the neurons in a delicate balance of complexity, majesty, and beauty. The process of dementia destroys these processes.

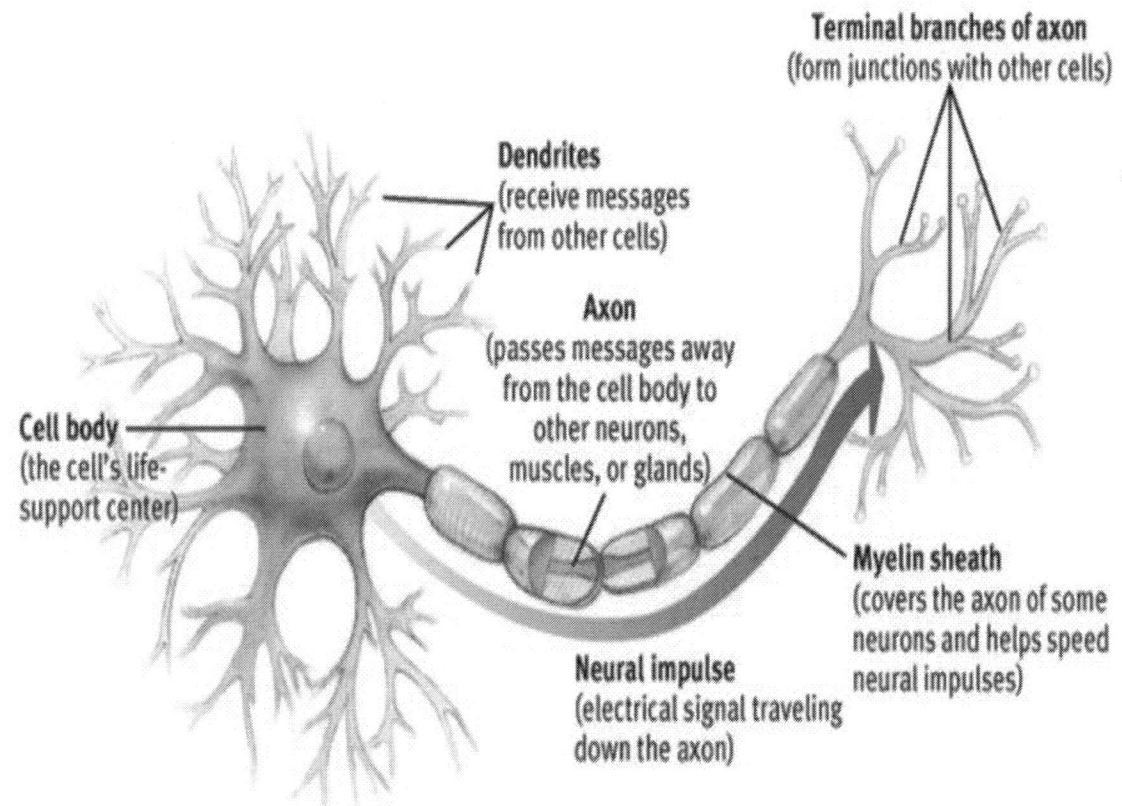

NOTES

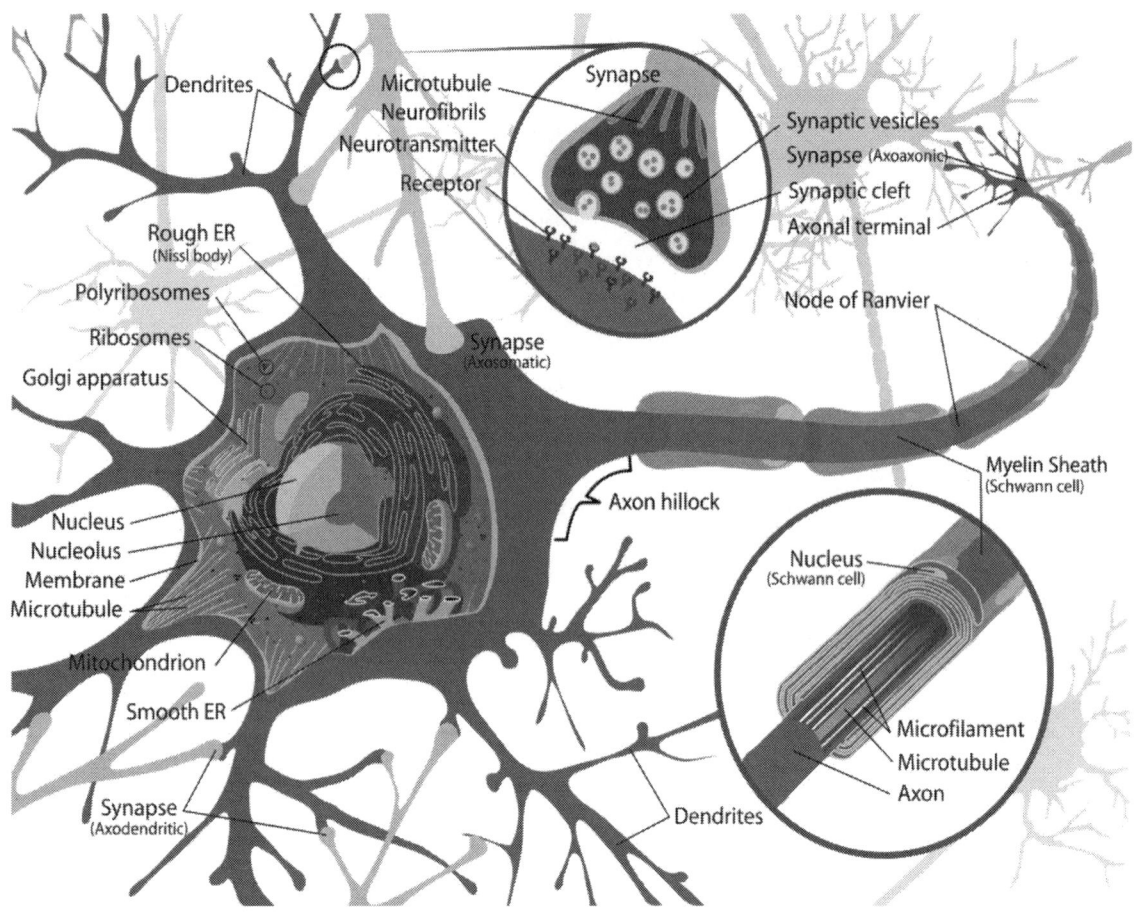

How is Memory Made?

Memory is made through a complex set of processes in the brain that are not fully understood. Certain parts have been identified as key to the process, but the formation of memory and the identification and manner of selecting where memories are stored in the brain are still being mapped out.

However, the hippocampus and the limbic systems must be undamaged for memory to be made and encoded or stored. In most forms of dementia, these areas are impacted early in the disease. Eventually, these critical brain structures are destroyed and have been removed from the brain cell by cell, until what remains is a space filled only with cerebral spinal fluid.

Memory formation begins at the moment of birth. The first person you met was your mother. When your father and mother left the hospital, they took you home. You began to learn the same things all humans learn. Names, family structures, social skills, language, religion, singing, cursing, and the Activities of Daily Living or ADLs.

Your first ADL was eating; your second ADL was a developmental milestone in humans. You transferred yourself from lying on your back to turning over on your stomach. Then you learned to walk by pulling up and balancing, then taking steps (ambulating.) You began to learn how to bathe, the most complex ADL. It takes about 10 years to learn this most difficult ADL safely and correctly. You were taught to toilet and in doing so how to control your bladder and bowels. Dressing and grooming rounded out your ADL education.

You attended school, learning more social skills and making friends. You learned reading, writing, math, games, music, driving, and dating. After graduating, you went to college, the military, or a job. You found a home, fell in love, and got married.

You became a parent, bought a house, continued your career, and aged from a young adult to a mature adult. You had children and taught them the same things you learned.

Those children gave you grandchildren and eventually great grandchildren joined your family. Along the way you buried grandparents and parents, finally arriving at being an older adult and retired.

Cells phones, flat screen televisions, and remote controls flooded our lives around 2005. Social media began, online life started, and common things around you became not so common.

And then there was a pandemic.

In most forms of dementia, memory begins to be erased in the reverse order it was learned, and your loved one can appear to be traveling back in time with their memories.

To help you understand what is happening to a Person with Dementia, think of every memory as a file of information and the brain as the file cabinet. People without dementia have cabinets that are organized and full. They are aware of the correct time, date, and place at any given moment.

In the Person with Dementia, the connections between the neurons are being destroyed. Proteins are clumping together or becoming tangles of filaments disrupting cell function internally. Some damage stops the cells from touching and communicating with each other. Other changes disrupt the ability of the cell to take in nutrition, causing it to starve to death. The destruction is massive and ultimately terminal for the Person with Dementia.

Nothing the Person with Dementia does is on purpose; it is all related to the damage occurring in her brain.

e

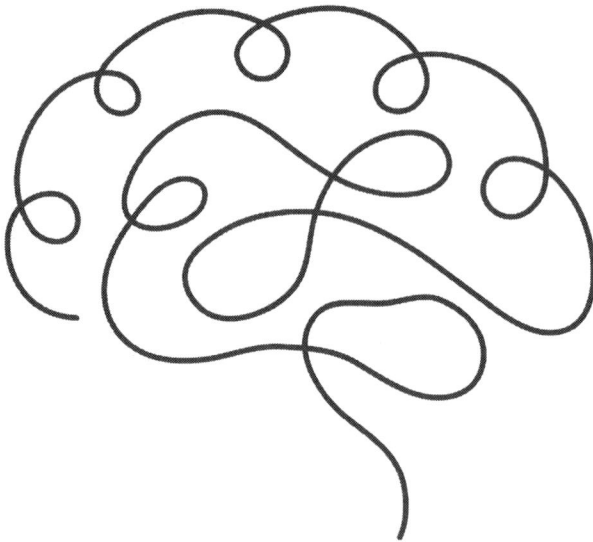

How Complex is the Brain?
- **Your brain has 100,000 miles of blood vessels. That's enough to go around the equator more than four times.**
- **The normal brain gets thicker and richer with dendritic growth as we age. We have neurons with dendrites several inches long.**
- **Dendrites continue to grow and add new tabs or spines allowing neighboring cells' axons to make new connections.**
- **Your brain is tightly folded to fit into the cranium. Unfolded, it would cover more than two square feet of space.**

Memory as a File Cabinet   NOTES

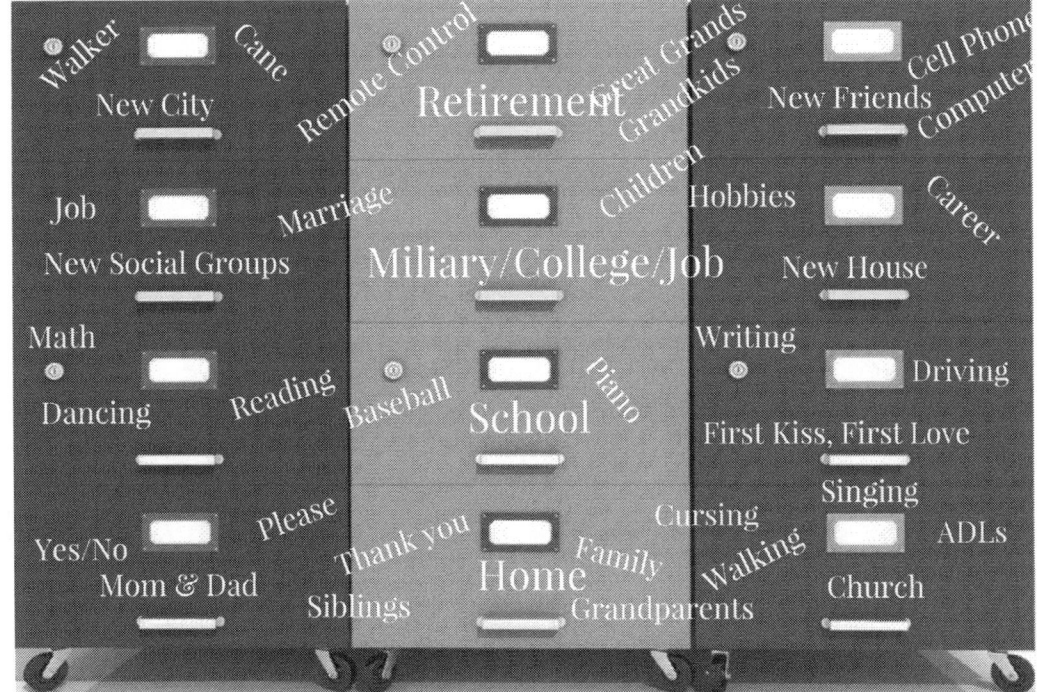

The File Cabinet exercise on page 48 will help you determine where your loved one's memories are currently filed. As you think about the Person with Dementia's lifetime, fill in each of the sections of the file cabinet with memories and people that would be present at that time in life. As you go up the File Cabinet, the ages associated with the files represent the skills and memories normally learned and made in that time of life.

Note when the death of parents or grandparents or other important family members occurred, because memories of that person stopped at that time.

Mark the current date at the top of the File Cabinet and underneath it, list the date the Person with Dementia thinks it is. The date the Person with Dementia believes it is also tells you where they are in their files. For example, if the year is 2030, but my mother insists the year is 1990, then I know her files from 1990 to the present time are heavily damaged.

Start with the Person with Dementia's birth date at the bottom of the file cabinet, fill in the things you know that person should remember. The bottom row represents the beginning of life and the memory process. Social skills, family,

Activities of Daily Living, speech, language, singing and cursing can be found here. This is the time of life for the infant, toddler, and child.

The second row represents what would be learned in school. What the person learned, who they knew, when they began to drive, date, etc.

The third row is the young adult and mature adult years. This is the time of the first house or apartment, college, a job or the military. This time could be new friends, marriage, and children.

The fourth row is the time of the elder or older adult. It includes the addition of grandchildren, great grandchildren, retirement, etc. The fourth row also includes new information such as social media, remote controls, cell phones, new family members, etc.

Once the file cabinet is filled, cross out the information or memory that is no longer in existence. In most forms of dementia, memory will move backwards toward the bottom row. The newest information in the brain is the first

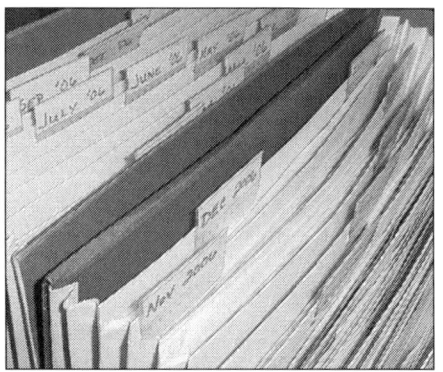
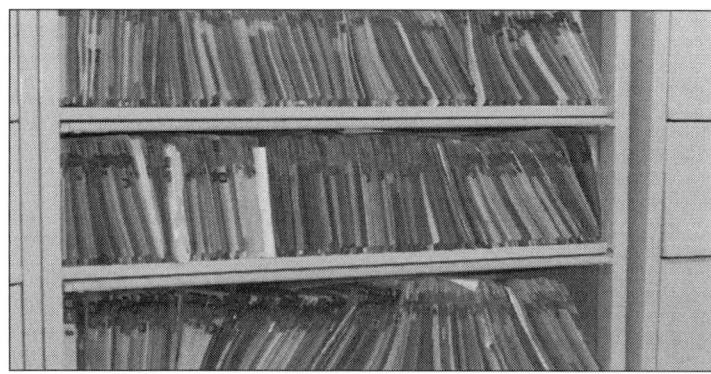

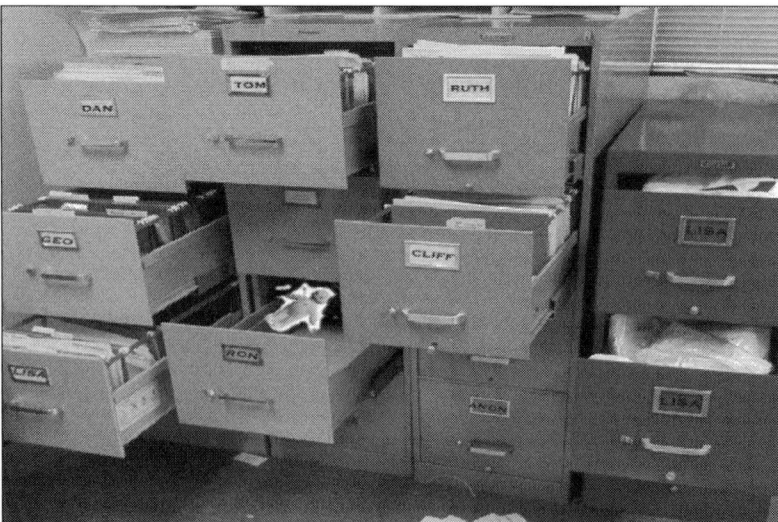

Some have very organized files.

Some do not.

information lost. In most forms of dementia, our oldest memories remain the longest.

Can you see now that the odd behavior and actions and words of a Person with Dementia are not purposeful? It is due to brain damage and which files remain intact. As memory is destroyed (most of the time in a reverse fashion), the Person with Dementia begins to acclimate herself to the place and people around her by using the remaining memories of the brain.

You, the daughter, can become the wife or the mother. You, the son, can become the father or the husband. The husband becomes a grandfather. The wife becomes the mother or grandmother. Adult children become lost or confused with siblings, cousins, or other family members. You are being matched to the files that still exist, to the files that make the most sense. It is most often that you physically favor the other person you are now being confused with.

Especially challenging for family and professional caregivers are memories that involve multiple marriages, stepchildren additions, blended families, etc. But eventually, the original family memories will be what remains.

Exceptions to this include persons with Vascular Dementias, Lewy Body Dementias, Parkinson Disease Dementias, Huntington's Dementias and Frontal Temporal Dementias (FTDs). Their brains are dying in a different order, so memory loss may or may not follow this retro-genesis pattern of loss.

Exercise

Fill in the file cabinet on the following page using the Person with Dementia's timeline of events. Then cross out the memories that appear to be missing. This will tell you which time of life is most present now. For example, if my mother doesn't remember being married and having children, grandchildren, and great grandchildren, then she must be in school. If she asks to go home and is frantic, then she is between the ages of three and nine, because that is where that emotional memory is held.

Date:	PWD's date:

NOTES

Older Adult Memories

Young Adult Memories

School Memories

Birth Date:

Early Memories

© 2022 Tam Cummings, Ph.D. tamcummings.com	48

Which telephone is the correct one?

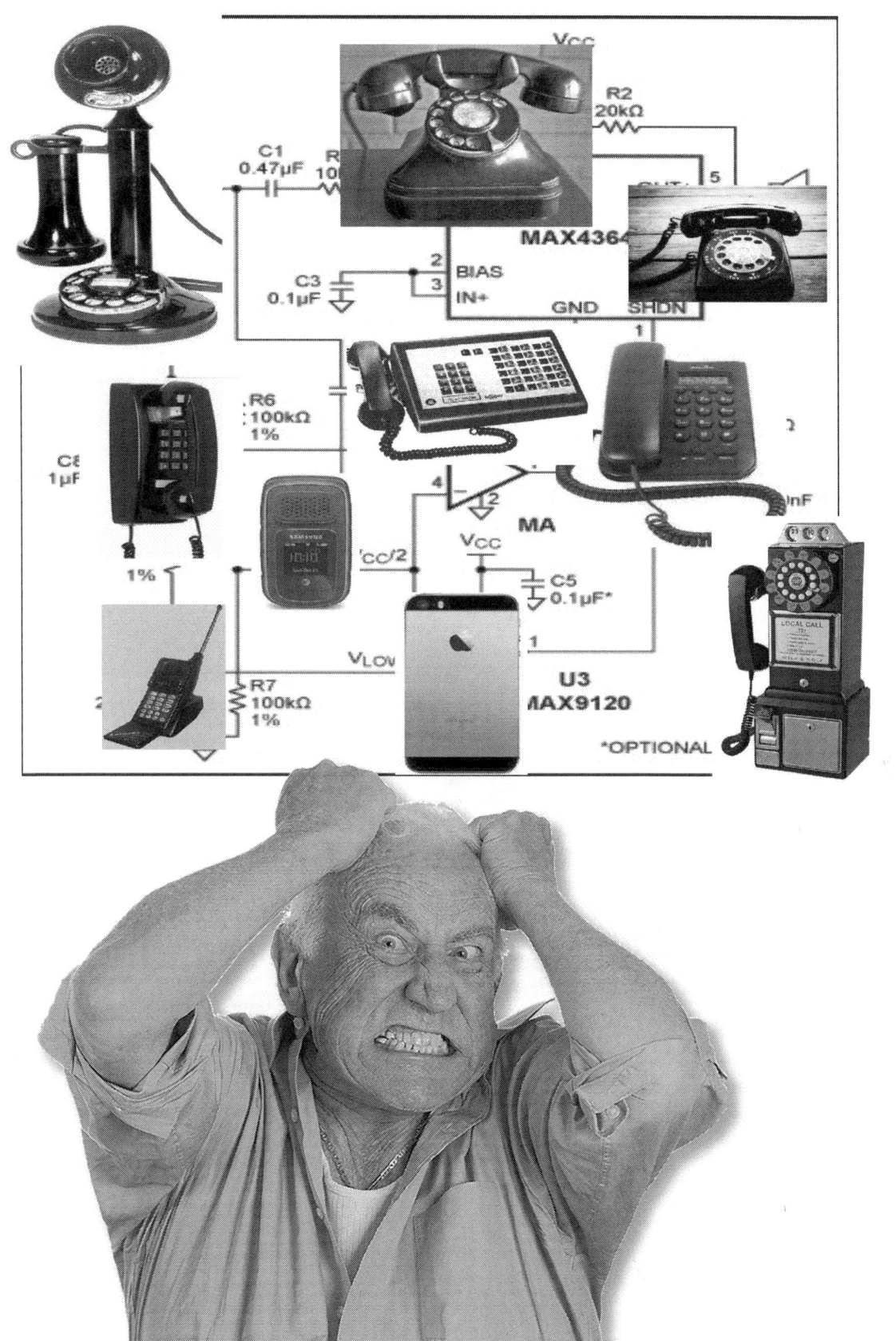

NOTES

Entertainment – books, then radio, finally TV, but not these new ones! NOTES

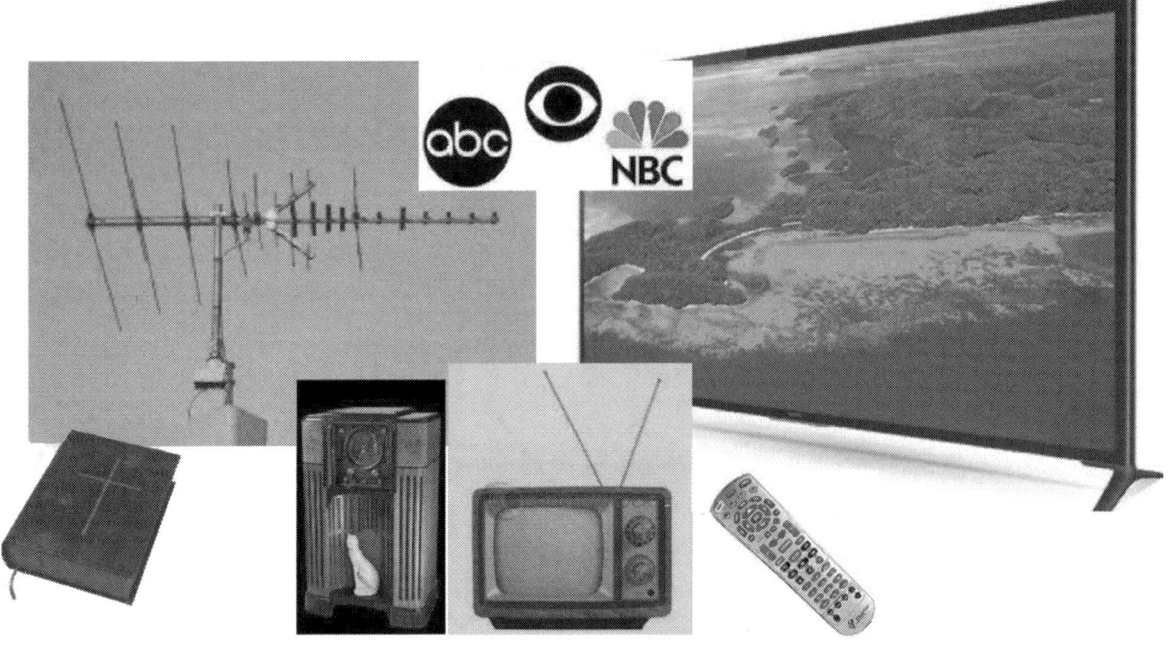

Bathrooms aren't all alike.

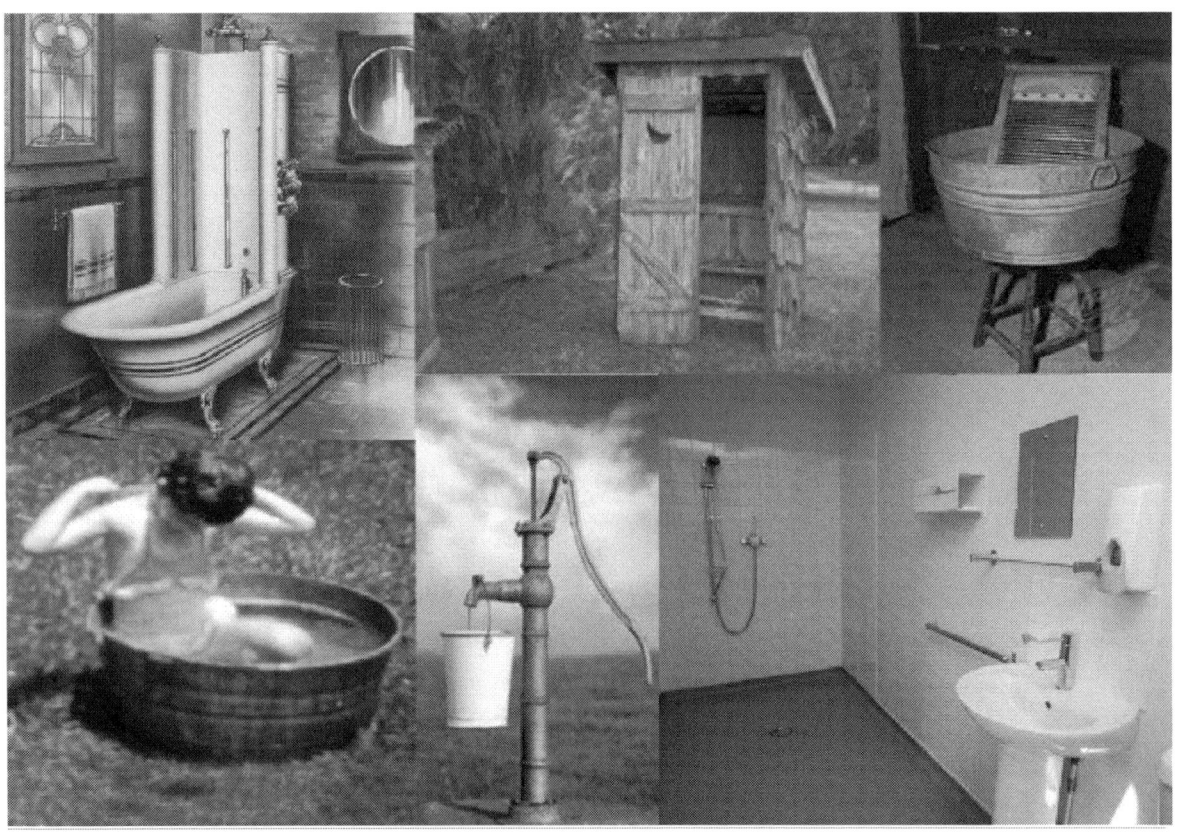

Can you do the laundry?

NOTES

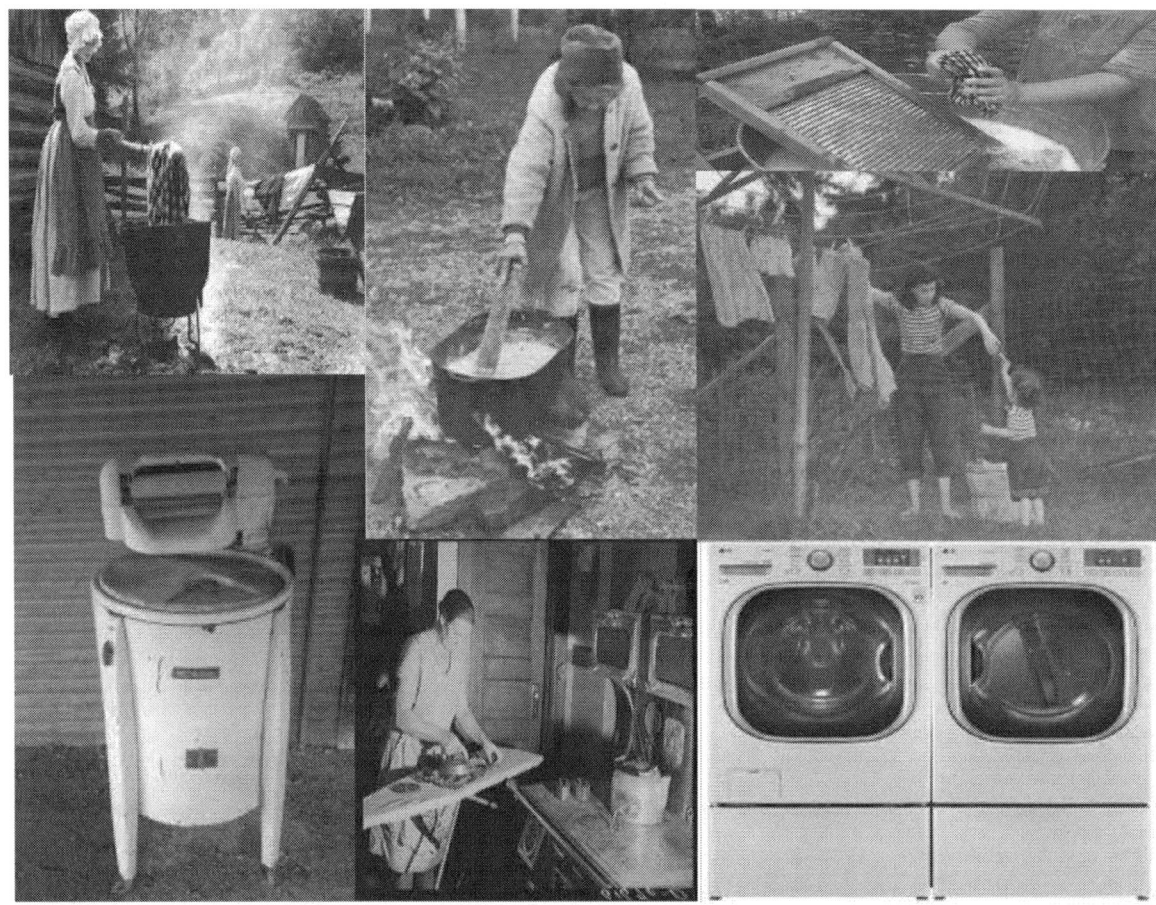

Conversation Tip
Never quiz the Person with Dementia. Questions should not be used in conversation. It is embarrassing to be asked "Do you know who I am?" or "Who is this person?" especially when the person doesn't recognize anyone. We don't enjoy people approaching us that way and neither do Persons with Dementia.

What could you try instead?

Try something like this:

> "Hi, I'm John, your youngest and most handsome son. I am better looking than your other children, Betsy and Jimbo and Rusty. I was always smarter and you always liked me more."

What a difference! This approach has used humor, named off other family members and given the Person with Dementia information he or she may be able to grasp. Make sure to train visiting friends and family members to do the same.

What the current available evidence says:

Most guidelines address the importance of communication, and it has been reported to be central to the interactions of persons, family members, and service providers. They are going back in time. Computers may not exist, iPad and iPhone don't exist. Siri and Alexa are strangers, as well as video games, facetime, etc. Our current language about them and any new invention makes no sense to a Person with Dementia as the disease progresses. Keep conversations within their reference.

- Use simple words and short sentences in a gentle, calm tone of voice.
- Avoid talking to the Person with Dementia at a reduced cognitive level or discussing the person as if the person is not there. Don't talk about things beyond their knowledge or frame of reference.
- Minimize distractions and noise to help the person focus on what you are saying. Remember their brain lobes — which translate everything around them — are damaged.
- Address the person by name, making sure you have his or her attention before speaking. Face the person with your eyes looking into their eyes and your face in their visual frame.

- Allow time for the person to respond independently. Be careful not to interrupt.
- If the Person with Dementia is struggling to find a word or communicate a thought, gently try to provide the word he or she is looking for.
- Try to frame questions and instructions in a positive way.
- When talking with the Person with Dementia, explain all procedures and activities in simple and straightforward terms to the person before performing them. If the task means moving a painful joint, prepare them and talk them through the action and apologize for causing any pain. Acknowledge the humanity in the human and display yours.
- Continue this conversation with each step, gently, slowly and with praise for leaning forward, lifting the arm, looking pretty in her sweater, etc. as you finish this component of the ADL of dressing. **If you should cause her pain, immediately apologize to continue to build the relationship.**

> *"Miss Margie, we are going to put on your sweater and keep you warm. Let's start on your right side. I know that your elbow hurts so I will be extra careful. You put your arm in the best you can, and I'll put the sleeve up for you."*

Remember the Person with Dementia may or may not be able to understand speech. If you have an accent, work on your phrasing and word pronunciation. It is vitally important to be understood.

Once I asked a lady if her mother was a nice cook and she almost flogged me because she heard me call her mother a "nice crook."

Don't forget that automatic "yes/no" responses remain until speech is lost and do not mean the person understands what "yes" means or what "no" means.

For specific conversations, turn off televisions, radio, music, cell phone, etc. The Person with Dementia's brain needs to be able to focus on the conversation. He or she begins to have difficulty filtering out background noise, so be aware of other sounds. This is due to damage in the temporal lobes.

Be prepared to take time, make eye contact, sit down, speak in short sentences, repeat information, repeat information, repeat information. **The very act of sitting in the Person with Dementia's presence, even for 10 seconds, often leaves the person feeling as though you have been sitting there for several minutes and therefore, you must be a friend. Who would you allow to assist you, a stranger, or your friend?**

Know the person's history. If you work with older generations, you should know American history: the presidents, the wars, aspects of the wars, like a Victory Garden, ration stamps, Axis powers, Allied powers, Vietnam, and Korea, etc. You should know songs and movies, television shows and stars, and popular sayings. Know the person's family, children, spouse, parents, grandparents, etc. Know the person's birthplace, family background, favorite foods, children's names, spouse's name, etc.

The brain of a Person with Dementia is being destroyed. It's nothing they asked for or wanted or deserved. It just happened. And this person is not refusing to do what you want, they simply can't understand everything. This is not a "use it or lose it" situation. This is a "doing the best I can" scenario. Dementias destroy the brain. The brain runs the body, and in the course of the disease, the body works less and less efficiently.

Watch the questions. To question Persons with Dementia is considered rude and cruel. People with Dementia are doing the best they can. In the beginning of Stage 5, it is thought the Person with Dementia can understand three out of four words. By the end of the disease, he or she understands no words, but still interprets tone and pitch and volume. Balance the decline with the knowledge that this is still an adult and should not be talked to as though he or she is a child. Sometimes the only communication skill needed is to sit quietly and hold a hand.

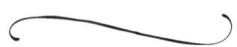

NOTES

Five Things to Remember

1. Memory means the ability to retain, recall or store (encode) information.

2. In medical terms, memory means the ability to transfer, ambulate, toilet, bathe, groom, dress, eat, use and understand language, and recognize yourself and others. People With Dementia lose the ability to do these things during the course of the disease as dementia destroys brain cells.

3. Memory is formed by the hippocampus and limbic areas of the brain. Once these areas are damaged or destroyed, the PWD cannot make any new memories.

4. Dementias destroy the brain's cellular structures and functions.

5. People with Dementia are not aware they are having cognitive challenges.

NOTES

Four
THE NINE COMMON DEMENTIAS

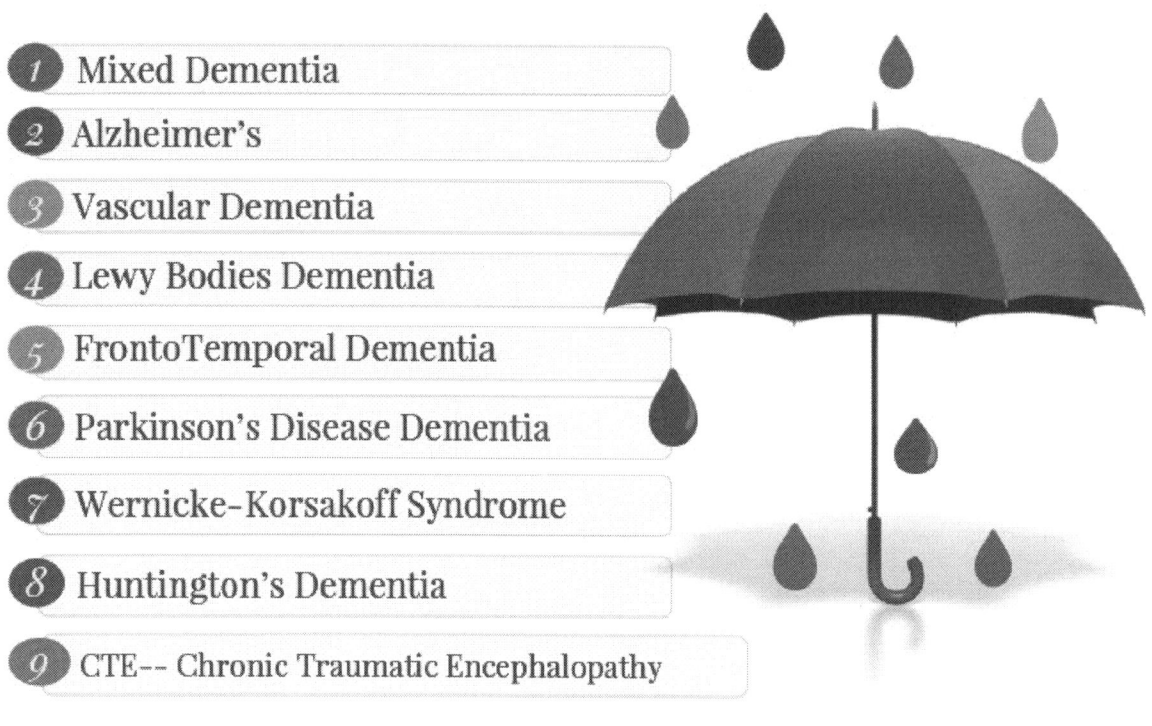

1. Mixed Dementia
2. Alzheimer's
3. Vascular Dementia
4. Lewy Bodies Dementia
5. FrontoTemporal Dementia
6. Parkinson's Disease Dementia
7. Wernicke-Korsakoff Syndrome
8. Huntington's Dementia
9. CTE-- Chronic Traumatic Encephalopathy

Dementia

Let's review now that you understand the functions of the brain lobes. Dementia is the umbrella term for a group of terminal brain diseases. To qualify as a dementia, the disease must affect two of the seven lobes of the brain.

There are four major and three minor lobes on each side of the brain. The disease must interfere with a person's ability to function, meaning to perform and complete the Activities of Daily Living (ADLs) and the Instrumental Activities of Daily Living (IADLs).

The disease must cause the loss of memory, which is all the accumulated information that makes you who you are. How you walk; how you chew food; how you greet others; how you appear; how you see yourself; your life, your personality, your family, education, skills, hobbies, experiences, loves, losses, births, and deaths — all are parts of memory.

Dementia is a progressive and terminal disease. The brain runs the body. A damaged brain cannot correctly operate or protect the body systems. People with Dementia fall and suffer from urinary tract infections (UTIs) because of brain damage.

At the end of dementia, the Person with Dementia doesn't recognize herself. She doesn't know her family. She is totally reliant upon others for care. She cannot use or respond to language; she cannot chew or swallow food properly. If her death doesn't come from a stroke or heart attack, her end will come from aspirating food into her lungs, developing pneumonia, widespread infection, and kidney failure (renal failure).

Forty-eight dementias have been identified, although a different set of classifications lists 108 dementias. These dementias have subsets and mutations and mixtures of different types. The largest of the dementia groups is Mixed Dementias, the second group is Dementias of the Alzheimer's Type.

Challenges for Caregivers and the Identification and Treatment of Dementias

- Early death of the caregiver due to stress and exhaustion
- Isolation of the caregiver
- No standardized or required testing to declare the diagnosis
- No clear path to care
- Lack of federal or state involvement to support care at home
- Prohibitive costs of care
- Risk of losing home or savings
- No medications for stopping the progression of the disease

Classifications of Dementias

People often leave confused after discussions with doctors due to the variation and complexity of dementias. The word "disease" has now been replaced by the word "dementia." Alzheimer's Disease is now referred to as Alzheimer's Dementia.

But the medical name/term is Dementias of the Alzheimer's Type or DAT. Vascular Dementia is now referred to as Dementias of the Vascular Type.

Currently, all dementias are classified as Major Neurocognitive Diseases, which more clearly addresses and describes what the diseases do to the brain. Translated, the name means neuro (brain) cognitive (ability to think, use memory, movement, language, etc.) disease. Dementias cause significant damage and eventually destroy the brain.

Dementias are also classified as either Dementias of the Alzheimer's Type and Non-Alzheimer's Dementias. Other descriptions used to distinguish dementias, or to give details about the disease, follow. Variations within types of dementias are called domains.

Secondary Dementia

This dementia develops as a peripheral, or secondary, condition to a pre-existing mental condition or illness. Progressive supranuclear palsy, a FrontoTemporal movement dementia, is an example of a secondary dementia.

Multiple Dementias

Research has shown it may be common for a Person with Dementia to have more than one form of the disease. The most common form of Mixed Dementia is the combination of Alzheimer's and Vascular Dementias.

Through new testing, along with information from longitudinal research, it appears there are multiple mixtures of Alzheimer's and any other dementia, for example, Lewy Bodies and Alzheimer's, Vascular and FrontoTemporal Dementia and Alzheimer's. Some people may have as many as four or five different forms of dementia.

Often, the professional caregiver's direct observation of behaviors begins to point doctors towards the realization that the Person with Dementia is struggling with multiple forms of dementia at once.

NOTES

Cortical Dementias

Damage begins primarily on the brain's cortex, or outer layer. The folds and turns of the outer layer function in part for language and memory. The gray matter of the brain is impacted. These dementias cause problems with memory, language, the ability to find the right word, thinking, and social behavior. Alzheimer's, Binswanger's Disease (Vascular Dementia form), FrontoTemporal Dementia (FTD), and Creutzfeldt-Jakob are cortical dementias.

Subcortical Dementia

The initial damage in these dementias occurs in the parts of the brain below the cortex and include more functional damage to the white matter of the brain. Huntington's, Parkinson's Disease Dementias, and AIDS Dementia Complex are subcortical dementias.

The ability to start activities and the speed of thinking are usually impaired, while forgetfulness and language are unchanged. Changes in personality, emotions and movements are noted, and in time there are memory problems.

Dementias Related to Sports

Chronic Traumatic Encephalopathy – Football Dementia and Soccer Dementia, Pugilistic Encephalopathy – Boxer's Dementia.

Inflammatory Disorder Dementias
- Multiple Sclerosis
- Vasculitis with or without Systemic Involvement
- Systemic Lupus Erythematosus
- Sjogren's Syndrome
- Sarcoidosis
- Bechet's Disease
- Non-Vasculitic Autoimmune Encephalomyelitis (NAIM)

Toxin Dementias
- Alcohol, Chemicals, Cigarette Smoke

Structural Pathology Dementias
- Malignant Tumors
- Benign Tumors
- Abscesses

Infection-Related Dementias
- Creutzfeldt-Jacob Disease
- HIV-Related Dementia
- Syphilis
- Whipple's Disease
- Herpes Encephalitis and other Viral Encephalitides
- Chronic Meningitis
- Progressive Multifocal Leukoencephalopathy
- Subacute Sclerosing Panencephalitis

Metabolic-Related Dementias
- B12 Deficiency
- Thyroid Disease
- Parathyroid Disease

Hereditary Dementias
- Early Onset Alzheimer's (EOA), Familial Alzheimer's Dementia (FAD)
- Huntington's Disease, Juvenile Huntington's Disease, and/or Huntington's Chorea
- CADASIL, and other forms of Vascular Dementias are known to be inherited.

Unusual Progressions in Dementia

For each form of dementia there can be severe, and most often, unexplained, or sudden declines in the health and cognition of the Person with Dementia. There are several factors to keep in mind as these events begin to occur. Any person with

NOTES

a dementia may suffer unnoticed seizures or mild stroke activity. These events are thought to be more commonly occurring during night sleep and therefore often go undetected because the change is subtle.

In dementia care it isn't the second, or third, or even the tenth stroke that may change the person's behavior. It's the stroke that tipped the balance in the brain's ability to function. Strokes alter the brain's overall structure and create noticeable changes. A Person with Dementia may have accumulated dozens of strokes over time with no one noticing a difference in behavior. Eventually enough damage occurs so that the overall effect catches up and others can observe the changes in the person's behavior and abilities.

There may have been an unwitnessed fall with a head strike. Remember, the brain is shrinking due to the loss of tissue. The dying cells are being removed from the brain as the body rids itself of dead or broken cells and proteins. The brain structure will eventually have a large amount of cerebrospinal fluid in the central ventricles and the brain may even be floating in cerebrospinal fluid.

Falls with strikes to the head can cause significant damage in just one fall because of the loss of tissue. The force of the fall and the force of the impact from the fall can have serious effects. The combined energy of a fall with a head strike causes the brain to shift back and forth inside the cranium.

Striking the front or rear of the head is medically referred to as a contrecoup strike. A significant blow to either the front or back of the head, combined with the energy or force from the fall, causes a bouncing effect in which the brain strikes the front and back of the cranium. These falls cause additional damage to the brain tissue as the brain moves and bounces within the space of the cranium. Sudden and dramatic changes that significantly advance the disease progress in the Person with Dementia can certainly be linked to falls with strikes or impact to the head.

Dementias are described medically as inflammatory diseases. Changes in the function of the brain-blood barrier, responsible for removing dead cells and broken proteins from the brain, may cause unusual changes to occur in the Person with Dementia as the ability to clean the brain diminishes.

NOTES

Another inflammatory effect can happen suddenly and usually disappears within a few days. The Person with Dementia begins walking bent at the waist to the right side of her body, or her body is at an odd angle and out-of-balance. She moves and walks with her body leaning sideways. She may not show an infection in blood or urine tests, and scans for stroke activity may be equally unproductive. In a few days she will straighten back up and walk the way she had previously. It is theorized that this is due to a sudden inflammation of the brain; however, she should be seen by a physician to determine next steps for care.

The inflammation occurs because the disease process eventually damages the blood-brain barrier. Normally this barrier protects the brain by preventing harmful bacteria, viruses, or other infections from entering the brain structure. The brain-blood barrier allows oxygen to pass through to supply the brain, along with glucose to provide nutrition.

Likewise, the barrier provides a way for the brain to safely clear out and dispose of toxic debris, such as broken beta-amyloid, twisted tau proteins, and assorted dead cell pieces. The buildup of these bits and pieces of cellular structure causes inflammation to occur due to their toxicity. The continued stress to the brain-blood barrier begins to cause vascular problems in the brain structure as well.

The Nine Most Common Dementias

Listed on the next page are the most common forms of dementia by order of occurrence as determined by the National Institutes of Health (NIH).

Each of the dementia forms has variations, additional domains, and can join each other forming a Mixed Dementia. These nine dementias are estimated to be 98 percent of all the dementias, given the rarity of most other forms.

Once you understand these nine dementias, remove the ones your loved one cannot have, and return to the physician with the dementias remaining on the list.

1. **Mixed Dementia**
2. **Dementias of the Alzheimer's Type**
3. **Dementias of the Vascular Type**
4. **Lewy Bodies Dementia**
5. **FrontoTemporal Dementia**
6. **Parkinson's Disease Dementia**
7. **Wernicke-Korsakoff Syndrome**
8. **Huntington's Dementia**
9. **Chronic Traumatic Encephalopathy**

Mixed Dementia

The name Mixed Dementia indicates the presence of more than one form of dementia.

Historically, Mixed Dementia is when a person suffers from both Alzheimer's Dementia and Vascular Dementia. How the disease presents in behaviors varies based on the location and severity of the stroke damage and the stage of Alzheimer's.

Recent research indicates more forms and variations of Mixed Dementias exist than were previously thought. Dementias of the Alzheimer's Type may join with any other form of dementia and Dementias of the Vascular Type can do the same, meaning you could see a great variation in behaviors and presentation of the disease.

Additional research also indicates some dementias may mutate or form variations of specific dementias. Dementias of the Lewy Bodies have shown dramatic shifts in presentations, leading to new questions about the progression and formation of dementias.

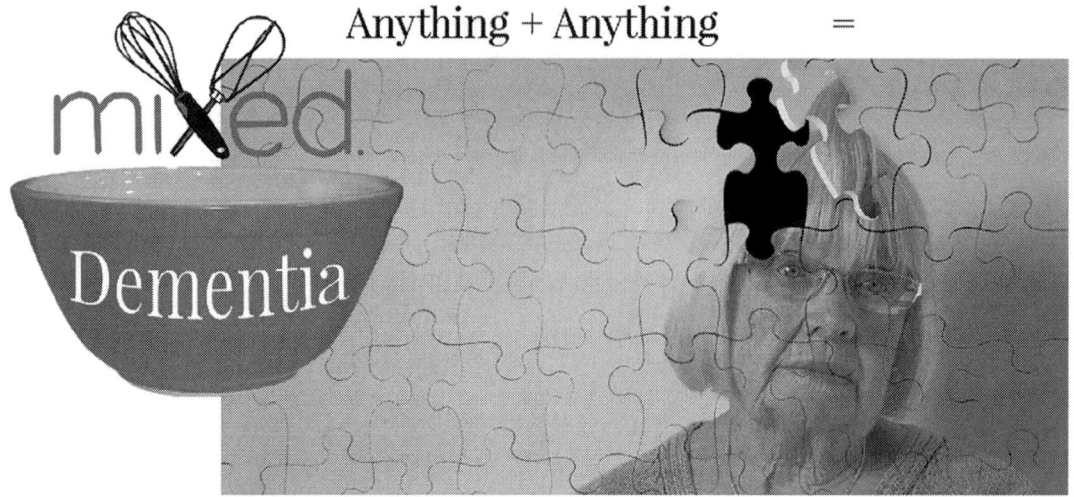

Alzheimer's + Vascular =
Alzheimer's + Anything =
Anything + Anything =
mixed Dementia

Order of Progression
- The location of stroke activity, along with identifying the stage of Alzheimer's Disease, helps determine the progression of Mixed Dementia. Identifying the features of additional dementias also helps determine the progression of the disease.

Anticipated Behaviors
- Behaviors of Alzheimer's and Vascular Dementias or any other forms of dementia can help pinpoint the disease progression.

Challenges
- Spotty areas in memory means doctors and family may not notice cognitive changes and thus can make disease progression difficult to diagnose.

Dementias of the Alzheimer's Type
Named for Dr. Alois Alzheimer.
- Early Onset Alzheimer's — Familial Alzheimer's Dementia (EOA-FAD) or Sporadic (estimated in 90 percent plus of cases)
- Down's Syndrome Alzheimer's
- Regular Onset Alzheimer's — variations with delusions, hallucinations, and/or persecutory beliefs, which may include aggressive, agitated, or anxious behaviors
- Late Onset Alzheimer's — variations with delusions, hallucinations, and/or persecutory beliefs, which may include aggressive, agitated, or anxious behaviors.

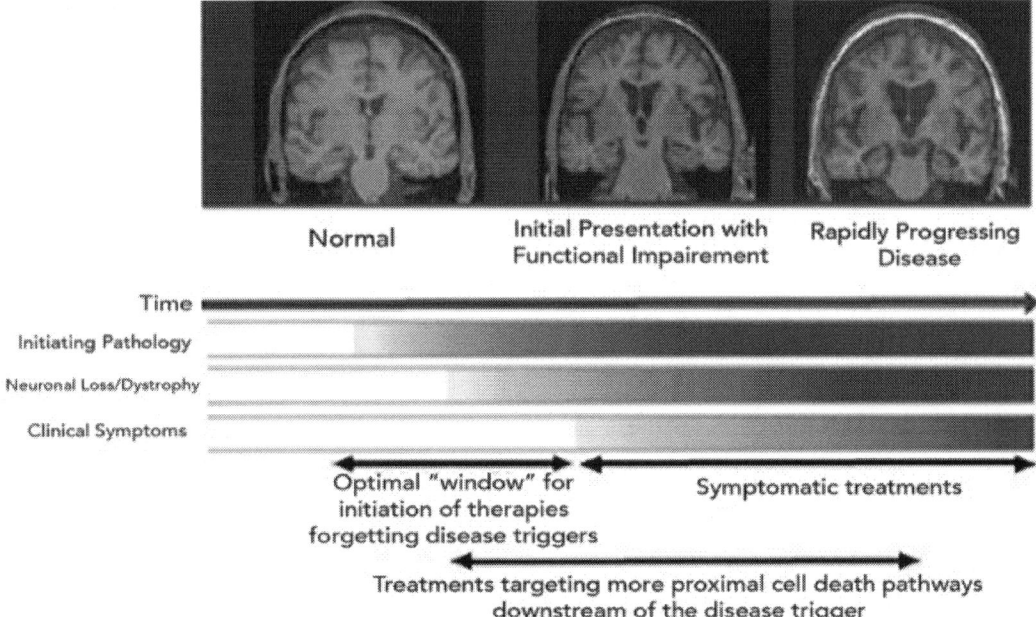

Alzheimer's Disease, except for EOA, begins as a cortical dementia on the surface of the brain. The entire brain is eventually impacted by the disease. Characteristic features of Alzheimer's Dementias are beta-amyloid plaques clumping between the nerve cells, impairing cellular function and neurofibrillary tangles of damaged tau proteins causing the cells to starve to death. It is not yet known if these two proteins start Alzheimer's or are a result of some other yet unidentified trigger.

Falls

- The most common fall is a fall backwards into the chair she is trying to rise from, with little damage to her body.

Early Onset Alzheimer's (EOA) Sporadic and Familial Alzheimer's Disease (FAD)

There are an estimated 500,000 persons in this country affected by EOA. The familial form strikes multiple persons within the family. This is not the 90-year-old-great-grandmother-form of Alzheimer's. This form attacks the young adult and mature adult, it attacks multiple family members, cousins, aunts, uncles, siblings, and one parent is also affected.

Most will display features between their 40s and 60s. There is typically a rapid and aggressive progression through the stages of the disease. Research suggests these families originated from a valley region of Germany and this is a genetic mutation shared through marriage.

The sporadic form of Early Onset Alzheimer's accounts for 90 percent of the cases. It may occur in a family with no history of dementia until a 35-year-old sister suddenly develops the disease.

In both forms, rapid and widespread atrophy occurs in all four lobes, followed by a decline in the medial temporal and parietal regions, before advancing to the cortical region. Research indicates there is a significant loss early in the disease of the brain's ability to metabolize glucose. The brain runs on glucose, so this is significant and possibly related to the rapid progression of the early dementias. Myoclonus, a form of muscle twitching and muscle spasms, are not uncommon in EOA. Death occurs typically within weeks of becoming bed bound.

This dementia's name is frequently misinterpreted by families. After visiting the doctor, the caregiver was told their loved one is in the early "stages" of dementia, meaning the disease is only beginning to show an impact visible to others.

Human nature and mistakes turn the word *stages* into the word *onset* and suddenly the diagnosis becomes *Early Onset Alzheimer's*, and the information families find about that disease doesn't make sense. Early Onset is the name of a disease and Early Stage tells you how advanced (early, middle, late) the disease is.

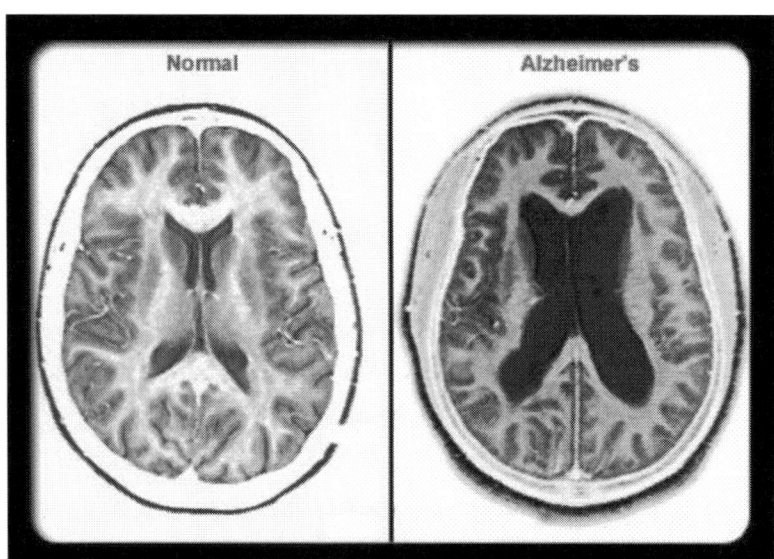

Down's Syndrome Alzheimer's

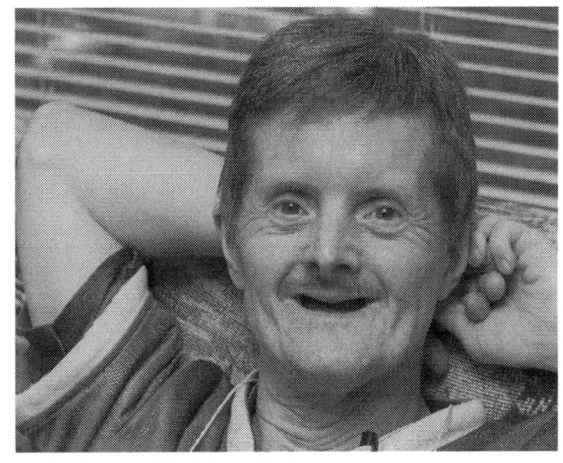

As early as the middle-to-late 40s, Persons with Downs' Syndrome begin to experience a significant buildup of plaques and neurofibrillary tangles in their brains. Spinal fluid testing shows enough plaque and tangles for a diagnosis of Alzheimer's Dementia, although symptoms may not show for ten more years. Alzheimer's neuropathology research indicates the disease accelerates between the ages of 40 and 50.

Cortical damage and white matter degeneration appear more profound in Downs' Syndrome. White matter contains bundles of neurons and microscopic blood vessels that feed the brain tissue. The accelerated aging found in Persons with Downs' Syndrome affects organs, structural and muscle systems. The impaired immune system is also a concern as the dementia progresses because a damaged brain cannot protect the body adequately from infection.

The onset of seizures and a distinctive and usually quite sudden refusal to perform the Activities of Daily Living (ADLs) are common behaviors. There is a marked decrease in the person's interest in hobbies or other activities, or a disappearance of the usual enthusiasm for previously enjoyed activities. The person will present a depressed state and a loss of effect on the face and in the voice. She may experience sleep disturbances, and exhibit increased sadness, fearfulness, or anxiety. Caregivers may witness irritability, uncooperative behavior, and even aggression from the Person with Dementia. Changes in coordinated movement are marked by a loss of balance and increased falls.

Nurses and physicians should be aware of depression, thyroid changes, chronic ear and sinus infections, vision loss, and sleep apnea. Staff should be alerted that persons with untreated sleep apnea experience multiple nightly events of oxygen loss to the brain. With each stoppage of breath, the person's heart comes close to collapse or an attack as it struggles to take in oxygen from the lungs, which have stopped working as breathing halts. The continual stress can cause blood clots in the vessels and lead to strokes. This can affect any person with sleep apnea.

Regular Onset Alzheimer's Dementia

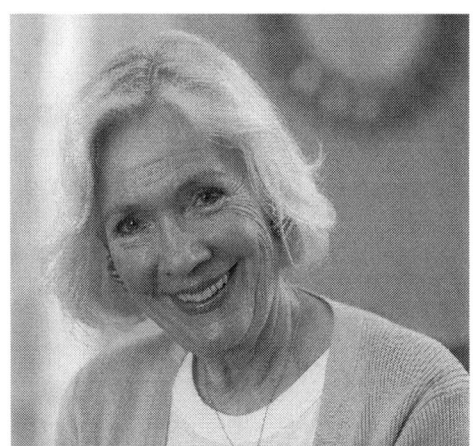

This dementia is generally thought of as persons showing symptoms in their 60s and 70s. Typically this person is unaware she is having memory problems, something called anosognosia. She therefore may become quickly frustrated and annoyed when she is corrected, or when errors are pointed out to her.

She may become momentarily concerned that people are talking about her or that she is in trouble. There are multiple forms of this dementia and individual mutations that can be expected.

This is an especially stressful dementia for the caregiver. As dementia progresses, loved ones see a person who loses the ability to plan for retirement, who will not know her grandchildren. They witness the death of a person who is categorized as young-old. However, for every Person with Dementia in this age group, it is estimated seven other people age normally.

There are multiple variations of Regular Onset Alzheimer's, including Atypical Frontal Variant Alzheimer's (fvAD) and Posterior Cortical Atrophy.

Late Onset Alzheimer's Dementia

This dementia occurs in people in their 80s and 90s who begin to show symptoms of cognitive changes. Again, they are typically unaware of the changes. It progresses more slowly than other forms of dementia. Due to the person's great age, death typically comes via a heart attack or stroke.

In gerontology, persons older than 85 are called the "Oldest-Old." In her eighties, she is in the ninth decade of life, and she has outlived other women born in her birth year by a dozen or more years.

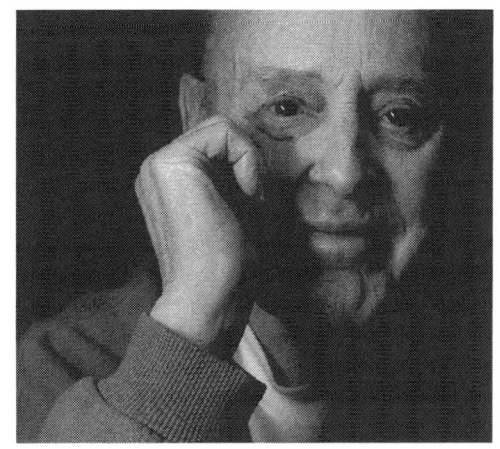

People with Dementia in their nineties have entered their tenth decade of life and are considered extremely old, frail, and fragile. At this great age they may still be strong, but it is vital to recognize they are frail and fragile. They can continue along with the disease in a stable state until a fall, or an illness, or infection, or hospitalization occurs. Then they fade quickly and die.

People in this age group are believed to have outlived all dementias except Late Onset Alzheimer's, Vascular Dementia or the combination called Mixed Dementia.

Progression of the disease

Typically, the disease begins on the outer area or cortex of the brain in the parietal lobe and eventually impacts the function of the hippocampus and limbic systems. These are the areas of the brain associated with learning new information.

Once these lobes become damaged, the person can no longer take new information in and lay down memory because the pieces of the brain that perform that function are damaged and eventually no longer exist in the brain's structure. At this point the Person with Dementia will rely and react using old information or memory that still exists in the brain.

While the spouse typically notices something is different in Stage Three of the disease, others, including family members, neighbors, co-workers, friends, physicians, and other professionals, often do not notice anything amiss until Stage Five of the disease. At this point, the hippocampus and limbic system are impacted, and the loss of short-term memory (STM) becomes apparent.

Signs that the disease has attacked the hippocampus will be indicated by repetitive questioning, sudden frustration, or angry outbursts without recognition of the behavior, and increased anxiety when away from familiar areas. Some families notice dementia for the first time in their loved one once she is taken on a trip. Removed from her regular landmarks and the familiarity of her bedroom and home, she will become increasingly agitated as the world around her makes no sense.

The reason her environment makes no sense is because her hippocampus is already damaged, and her brain can't figure out what is happening around it. The disease will typically progress from the hippocampus and limbic system to the temporal lobes, then to the frontal and occipital lobes, and finally the parietal lobes are impacted. The cerebellum and brain stem are damaged at the end of the disease.

The spouse will typically notice a change in behavior in Stage Three, but may be chastised for pointing out cognition changes, behavioral changes, or odd and unusual bursts of anger or anxiety. In Stage Four of the dementia, the adult children and friends and neighbors begin to suspect dementia.

For caregivers in urban areas, Stage Four can isolate them from their usual social circle. This is a process called Urban Isolationism. Friends stop calling or dropping by. Invitations to dinners, parties, golf, bridge, poker, coffee, etc., dry up as others react to the stigma or fear of dementia.

It is not unusual to meet a family caregiver completely cutoff from society as caregiving demands slowly exhaust him. Therefore, it is critical for caregivers to find and attend a caregiver support group as one way to deal with the stress and isolation.

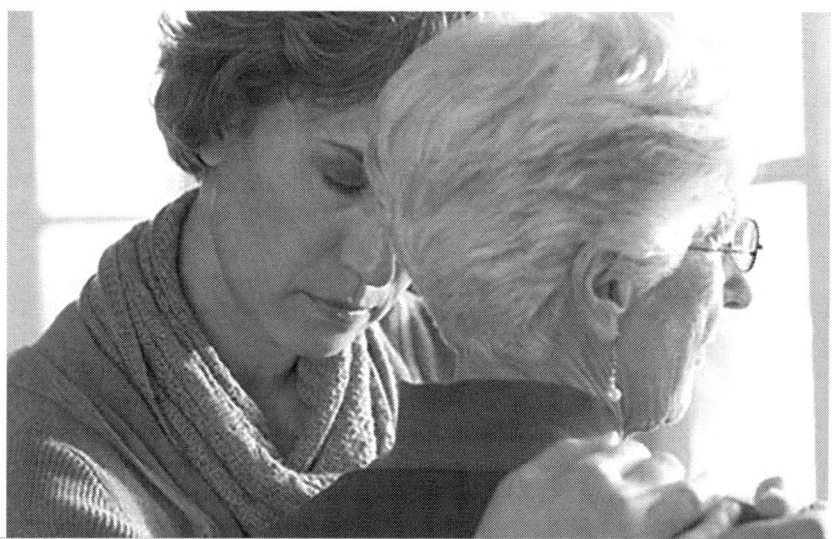

Stages Five, Six and Seven are also called the Terminal Stages or the Late Stages because death will occur in one of these stages for most people. Most persons aren't diagnosed until Stage Five of the disease, which leads to the statistic that people die within three to five years of the diagnosis.

The loss of short-term memory (STM) is noticed first, followed slowly, eventually, years later, by the loss of long-term memory (LTM). These two forms of memory may be separated by a decline that may last as long at 15 years following the diagnosis. However, most persons are not diagnosed with any dementia until Stage Five of the disease.

This is typically the stage when a family caregiver can convince the person to see a specialist, or when the family practitioner is alerted to memory problems. By Stage Five, there is global damage occurring in the brain and a significant loss of brain volume or brain tissue can be expected. It is estimated that at the Stage Five diagnosis, most people have already lost a half-pound or so of brain tissue and can still function and possibly fool an unskilled professional.

Behaviors will vary based on the progression of the disease and the presence of other medical conditions or other dementias. Visually, persons may experience illusions, misperceptions, and misidentifications, rather than hallucinations.

Challenges
- Death of the caregiver as a result of stress and exhaustion.
- Isolation of the caregiver.

NOTES

Dementias of the Vascular Type
Named for the Vascular System

Domains:
- Multi-Infarct Dementia, cortical or subcortical
- Binswanger
- Subcortical Vascular Dementia
- Amyloid Angiopathy
- Strategic Infarct-related Dementia (SID)
- CADASIL – Inherited
- Mixed Dementia and variations
- White Matter Disease
- Gray Matter Disease

Types of Strokes
Ischemic
- Clots that reduce blood flow
Hemorrhagic Stroke
- Blood vessel ruptures
Transient Ischemic Attack (TIA)
- Temporary blockage

Vascular Dementia may be caused by strokes, atherosclerosis, endocarditis, or amyloidosis. Structural damage to brain tissue can also be caused by blocked arteries, blood clots, or internal hemorrhaging.

Falls
- Common falls occur when trying to stand and move. This PWD frequently falls forward, landing on her face, elbows, and knees.

Strokes

Strokes can occur anywhere in the brain. The sneaky one is the silent stroke, often written off as "normal aging ischemic damage" by radiologists in MRI reports but considered by neurologists and gerontologists to be anything but "normal aging."

All strokes vary based on the type, size, causation, and location of the attack in the brain. Recovery from strokes is also based on the area of the brain and the size, type, and frequency of the stroke.

Migraine headaches are not uncommon as a symptom along with transient ischemic attacks or TIA strokes, but migraines do not mean a person is having a stroke.

Transient Ischemic Attacks (TIA)

Commonly called mini-strokes, baby strokes, tiny strokes, pen point strokes, these strokes typically last only a few moments. The clot is tiny and usually the brain recovers quickly. But the cumulative effect of years or decades of TIAs leads to Multi-Infarct Dementia or Multiple Stroke Dementia.

Ischemic Stroke

Ischemic strokes are caused by embolic clots that reduce blood flow as the clots move through the blood vessels. These clots originate elsewhere in the body and travel to the brain with the flow of blood, eventually reaching a blood vessel too small to allow the clot to pass, and the ischemic stroke occurs. Thrombotic clots are clumps of blood cells that form within the small brain arteries. Eventually the clot blocks blood flow and causes the stroke to occur.

Large Vessel Strokes

Large vessel strokes affect greater areas of the brain. Features include substantial swelling or bleeding in the brain, which may require surgery to open the cranium to relieve pressure. This would typically be a hemorrhagic stroke.

Silent Strokes

Silent strokes occur in the internal capsule of the brain. Activity on the left side of the brain affects the right side of the body and activity on the right side of the brain affects the left

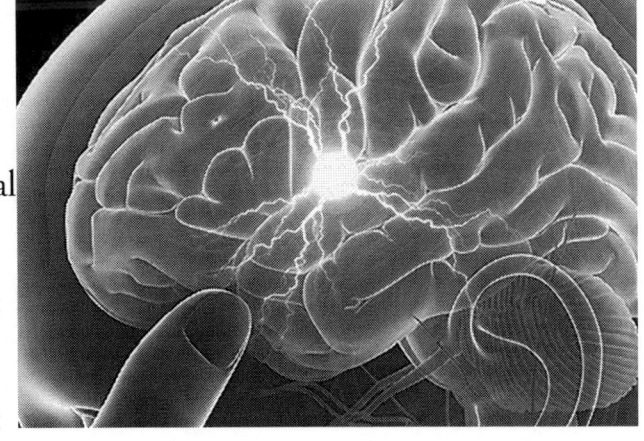

side of the body. The common causation of these strokes is the blockage of small blood vessels.

The internal capsule allows the cerebral cortex and areas of the brain stem to communicate. These connections allow physical movement and perception of sensory information (the five senses). Damage in this area means the arms, legs, trunk, and facial movements become impaired.

Binswanger's Disease

This dementia, Binswanger's Disease, begins in the early 40s and death typically occurs within five years. Cerebrovascular lesions in the deep white matter of the brain cause a loss of memory, mood changes, abnormal blood pressure readings, and an unsteady gait. Falls are anticipated early in the disease. This is a very aggressive dementia due to the young age of the person.

CADASIL

CADASIL is one of the hereditary dementias that also begins to show features in the late forties. Again, because of the age of the person, the disease process is quite aggressive. Death is usually within five years of diagnosis. Cerebral autosomal dominant arteriopathy with subcortical infarct and leukoencephalopathy (CADASIL) is a stroke dementia.

White Matter Disease

White matter disease is the tissue in the brain composed of microscopic blood vessels and bundles of nerves fibers. These bundles of nerves connect the brain to the spinal cord. The millions of fibers are covered by a fatty tissue called myelin sheath. This sheath provides insulation and protection for the nerves. The color of the myelin is what gives this area of the brain its name. Myelin speeds up signals between cells, allowing the brain to quickly assess a situation and respond.

White Matter Hyperintensities means the MRI scan is showing bright white areas, indicative of some type of brain injury. Decreased blood flow would indicate **white matter leukoaraiosis**. There might also be a diagnosis or conclusion of **non-specific white matter changes**, indicating no causation can be identified completely. Other causes of white spots could be TIAs (transient ischemic attack), multiple sclerosis, lupus, B12 deficiency, brain tumor, HIV, or Lyme Disease.

Gray Matter

Gray Matter is the area of the brain comprised of the neuronal cell bodies, glial cells, dendrites, myelinated and unmyelinated axons, synapses, capillaries. This is where the bulk of memory is contained. Again, the name comes from the color of the cells.

Anticipated Behaviors
- Problems with short-term memory
- Wandering or getting lost
- Laughing or crying at inappropriate times (Psuedobulbar Effect)
- Trouble concentrating
- Trouble managing money
- Aggressive behavior
- Inability to follow instructions
- Loss of bladder or bowel control
- Hallucinations
- Nighttime wandering
- Depression
- Incontinence
- One-sided body weakness
- Falls to the face, knees, and elbows or to the weak side of the body.

Challenges

- Death of the family caregiver due to stress.
- Increased chance of aggressive or highly agitated behaviors.
- Typically, the person has a history of high blood pressure or other cardiovascular disease.
- Risk factors are smoking, high cholesterol, diabetes, heart disease, inactivity, obesity, and inherited factors. African Americans and Hispanic Americans also have a higher risk factor for Vascular Dementia.
- Vascular Dementia's risk increases with the presence of atrial fibrillation, previous strokes, heart failure, cognitive decline prior to stroke, high blood pressure, diabetes and atherosclerosis, excess alcohol consumption, poor diet, and little to no physical activity.
- Catching vascular disease early, and diet and exercise make for a better prognosis.
- Family may have gone from having a normally aging person to a completely demented person from one stroke.

Dementias with Lewy Bodies (LBD)
Named for Dr. Frederic Lewy

Domains:

- Diffuse Lewy Bodies
- Cortical Lewy Bodies
- Parkinson's and Lewy Bodies
- Lewy Bodies and Parkinson's
- Dementia with Lewy Bodies
- Mixed Alzheimer's and Lewy Bodies
- Mixed Vascular and Lewy Bodies
- Mixed Lewy Bodies and FrontoTemporal Dementia

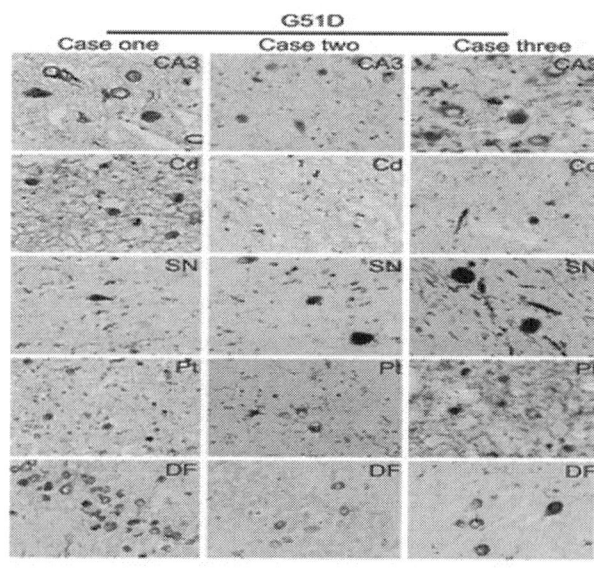

Area(s) of the Brain

Lewy Bodies proteins begin to form inside the brain's nerve cells. These abnormal deposits of the protein alpha-synuclein prevent the cell from functioning properly. Eventually, the disease may impact the hippocampus and limbic system. Symptoms may begin between the ages of 60 and 80. It is currently believed more males than females develop this dementia.

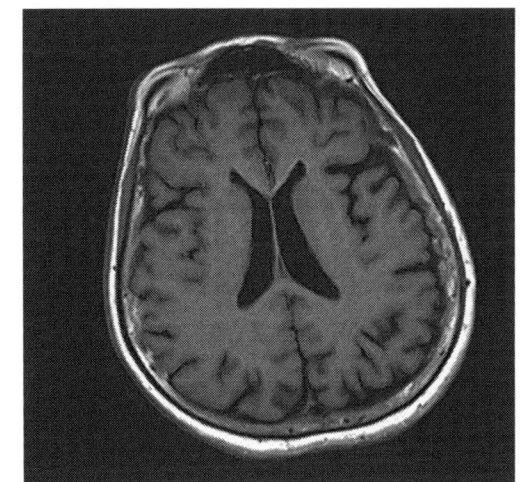

Falls

- Common falls are distinct and due to a sudden loss of consciousness. This person will stiffen like a plank and fall forward landing on her face. Or she may stiffen and fall backwards cracking the crown of her head. Parkinson's Disease Dementia falls are very similar to Lewy Bodies falls.

Progression

In a variation from the normal behavioral progress on the Dementia Behavioral Assessment Tool (DBAT), persons with LBD may accuse caregivers or family members or theft or sexual infidelity in Stage Three rather than Stage Five. Mild mannered husbands may begin to fixate on sexual activity and pressure the wife for intercourse, even scheduling dates and times. He may also ask for medication for erectile dysfunction, which adds to the challenge of care and the wife's stress.

Persons with LBD also may experience sudden and severe depression in Stage Three rather than late Stage Five. He may have moments or days of great confusion and frustration as his brain struggles with the change in the protein alpha synuclein.

As this protein begins to alter its function, and it begins to stay in the brain and its levels begin to build. This stops the brain from making the correct amounts of the chemicals acetylcholine and dopamine.

Acetylcholine affects memory and learning in brain function. Dopamine is a chemical that affects movement, moods, and sleep.

The visual hallucinations may appear in Stage Three, along with sudden changes in alertness, attention, and cognition. A slowness in movement is noted and gait changes include difficulty walking and rigidity.

This group is very sensitive to medications and should not receive anti-psychotics.

Anticipated Behavior

- Some symptoms of LBD can be similar to Alzheimer's Dementia.
- These include impaired memory, poor judgment, confusion, and depression. Anxiety and delusions may also be present, especially when cognition shifts intermittently. (Delusions are beliefs that are not real.)
- Delusions may include a sexual component and current news events. "My wife is having sex with the president on his plane but tomorrow when she goes to meet him on his plane, the plane will fall out of the sky."
- Or the delusion may stay closer to home with the wife accused to infidelity with everyone connected with this person, including the mailman, the doctor, the trash guy, the lawn man, the handyman, etc. REM sleep behavior begins (kicking or punching in sleep).
- Trouble falling asleep, restless leg syndrome, sleeping through the night then napping for hours the next day are also possible symptoms.
- Constipation not related to diet or medication, a shuffling gait, an inability to stand up straight, shaking, and increasingly dangerous falls are also noted. Perhaps best recognized by professional staff are the presence of hallucinogenic behaviors.
- Hallucinations are things a person may see, hear, smell, taste or feel that are not real. Common examples include seeing children.
- Seeing and knowing bad people are trying to kill you and one of those bad

people may be the son or daughter or another family member.
- Visual and tactile sensation of spiders, rats, snakes, and bugs crawling on you and biting you.
- Seeing the spouse or caregiver having sex with multiple people.

Challenges
- Death of the family caregiver due to the stress of care
- Death occurs five to eight years after diagnosis and usually involves complications from immobility
- Swallowing difficulties, chokes that lead to pneumonia, sepsis, renal failure
- Falls
- Poor nutrition
- Pneumonia
- The person is aware at times of what is happening
- The person may progress from merely being unsafe, but ambulatory, to being bed bound within days.
- Death typically follows within a few weeks or days.

FrontoTemporal Dementias
Named for Frontal and Temporal Lobes

Domains
- Behavioral Variant FTD (bvFTD)
- Pick's Dementia
- Corticobasal Degeneration (CBD)
- Progressive Supranuclear Palsy (PSP)
- FTD with Motor Neuron Disease or FTD with ALS
- Nonfluent/Agrammatic Variant Primary Progressive Aphasia
- Semantic Variant Primary Progressive Aphasia
- Logopenic Variant Primary Progressive Dementia
- FTD with HIV/AIDS
- FTD in any form with Dementia of the Alzheimer's Type (DAT)

NOTES

Area(s) of the Brain

The behaviors specific to areas of the frontal and temporal lobes determine which of these dementias a person has. The degeneration of nerve cells in these two sets of lobes and the accumulation of the tau protein and the protein TDP-43 cause damage to the brain. Some people have shown abnormal tau-filled lobes as well.

The average age of onset occurs between the 50s and 60s. The duration of the FTDs is between two and eight years. In these dementias, memory is functioning for a long time because the disease impacts the hippocampus and limbic systems later. But the areas of the brain that are affected mean we can expect to see significant changes in the person.

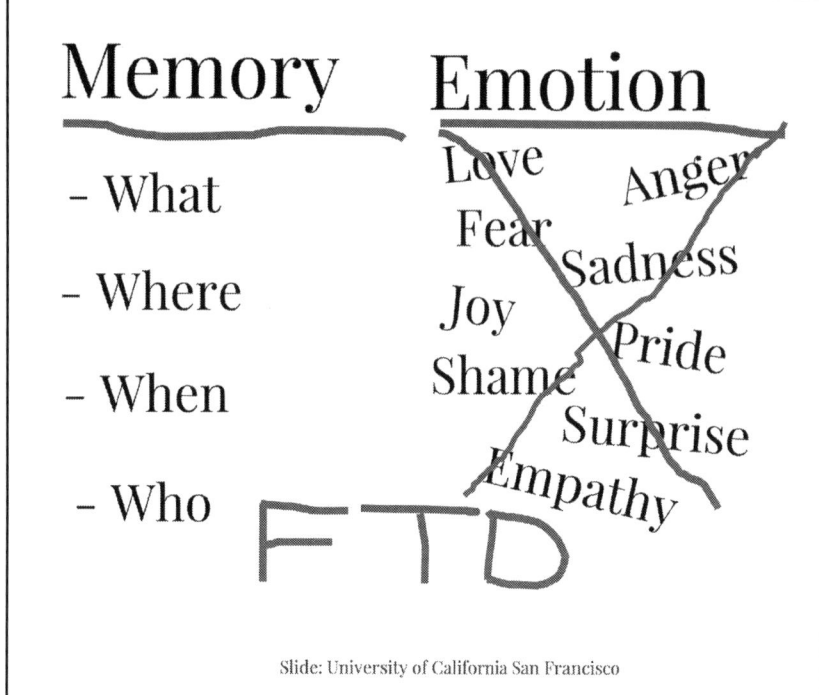

Slide: University of California San Francisco

Falls

- This population has unique falls. The movement disorder means FTDs are usually wheelchair bound early in the disease and may fall attempting to get up.
- FTDs become bent at the waist in the final stages of the disease. They suffer repeated falls with head strikes, which cause additional damage to the brain, due to the way the body can no longer stand and move normally. They will not keep helmets on, and falls can occur throughout the day.

Behavioral FrontoTemporal Dementias
Behavioral Variant FTD (bvFTD)

These persons display everything from apathy to a change in personality, loss of social boundaries and conduct, sexual inhibition, impulsive behavior, and craving sweets or certain foods or alcohol. It is not unusual to find that this person is only correctly diagnosed after being arrested for shoplifting.

Damage in the frontal lobes means there is a disconnect between the action and the consequence, so this person walks out of a store with no thought of hiding his actions, because he is not aware he has done anything wrong.

It is not unusual that this person has become estranged from his family as he will not appear ill but seems rather uncaring and unloving towards them. It is not unusual for this person to be recently divorced as the wife and children have left due to the unemotional responses from the husband/father.

More than half of the families of persons with FTD have no family history of these dementias. This person typically has a rapid decline towards the end of life.

Pick's Dementia
Named for Dr. Arnold Pick

Pick's Dementia has an average onset of symptoms in the person's mid-fifties. The Pick's Bodies are abnormal collections or the buildup of tau protein. Slow, steady, and progressive deterioration in behavior, personality or language can occur.

Behaviors include impulsivity, obsessive-compulsive behaviors, abrupt mood changes, unusual loss of social boundaries (may take off her clothing or masturbate in public) and demonstrate a lack of empathy.

Failure to understand financial outcomes can mean this person gives away her money without comprehending the consequences of being broke. When walking through the community, she may appear to "run over" other residents.

This is related to her impaired vision and care should be taken to protect her from residents angry about being knocked down and to protect residents from being walked into or being knocked down. From the loss of ambulation to becoming bed bound, death can occur in just a few weeks or months.

NOTES

Movement FrontoTemporal Dementias
Corticobasal Degeneration (CBD)

The presentation of this dementia may appear suddenly with an unexpected and detrimental onset. The disease causes a loss of nerve cells in the cerebral cortex and basal ganglia areas of the brain. The first symptoms may involve the motor system of the body or issues with cognition (difficulty with math is common) or both.

Symptoms also include Parkinsonian features such as poor coordination, muscle rigidity, and shaking. It also includes features of all late-stage dementias such as difficulty with speech, trouble swallowing, and memory loss.

This dementia is frequently misdiagnosed as Alzheimer's, Parkinson's Disease Dementia, Progressive Supranuclear Palsy (PSP, another of the FTDs), or Lewy Bodies Dementia. Due to the same areas of the brain being affected and similar behaviors and movements, physicians may confuse the diseases. The varied symptoms often lead to the correct diagnosis.

An estimated 40 to 60 percent of this group will develop alien hand syndrome, a condition in which one hand is not seen as controlled by the person. In other words, the person does not seem to be aware that the hand is there and is a part of their body. They are not able to identify the hand or rings on the hand. The brain is not able to find the hand. The brain is not aware the hand is there. The hand may react to stimuli, or it may not. Ideomotor apraxia (the inability to have coordinated muscle movement) may be seen in the hands and arms, or in the lower limbs causing walking challenges.

One foot may appear to be stuck to the floor, causing stumbling and falls. The fingers and hands may be unable to perform fine motor movements. This person may decline rapidly from Stage Six to Stage Seven and death may occur from choking, which then leads pneumonia, or another severe infection leading to sepsis and kidney failure (renal failure).

NOTES

Progressive Supranuclear Palsy (PSP)

This dementia causes issues with coordinated movement, gait, and balance. The hallmark feature of PSP is a progressive inability to coordinate eye movements. Related to the FTDs and Parkinson's groups, the features of this dementia also include depression, social and behavioral dysfunction, apathy towards life, hobbies, others, and depression. Generally, a noticeable cognitive decline does not occur.

The face is masked and immobile, and she will have difficulty with swallowing (dysphasia), making speech, and balance. The slowed and stiff gait increases her risk of falls.

This person may also exhibit embarrassing behaviors in social settings, saying or doing inappropriate things. She will appear to have no facial emotion or emotional blunting. To outsiders, she may appear indifferent to others. The brain stem, which controls balance and eye movements, is atrophied, and contains deposits of an abnormal form of tau protein. The decline to death is typically rapid.

> **Pseudobulbar Effect** is when a person suffers forced crying or laughing that is uncontrolled. It is not uncommon in PSP dementia and many other forms as well. Remember, even if the PWD is laughing, it is not funny. Life is not pleasant for the Person with Dementia. She is not in control of her behavior, and it causes increased anxiety if not treated.

FTD with Motor Neuron Disease, also known as FTD with ALS

This dementia affects approximately 10 to 15 percent of the people with FTD. The muscles atrophy, are stiff, and the person has difficulty with fine motor movements. She may experience fine muscle twitches and cramps.

The arms and legs on one or both sides of the body may be affected, and eventually more motor system functions will become impaired. Shortness of breath, falls, muscle twitches, exaggerated reflexes, and difficulty swallowing with coughing due to food or saliva in the windpipe. Death occurs from aspiration pneumonia, sepsis, and kidney failure (renal failure).

Communication in FrontoTemporal Dementias
Primary Progressive Aphasia (PPA)

This dementia affects a person's ability to speak, read, write, and understand what others are saying. Swallowing safely becomes a concern near the end of the disease. Death is typically from aspiration pneumonia, sepsis, and kidney failure (renal failure). There are three clinical subtypes of PPA.

Nonfluent/Agrammatic Variant Primary Progressive Aphasia

A person with this dementia form begins to have a loss or deterioration in her ability to produce speech. At first, her speech becomes hesitant, and she begins to 'talk around" the missing words, then she begins to talk less and less, eventually becoming mute. Behavior and personality changes will not occur until the late stages of dementia (Stages Five, Six and Seven). Difficulty swallowing leads to death by aspiration pneumonia, sepsis, and kidney failure (renal failure).

Semantic Variant Primary Progressive Aphasia

This person demonstrates a progressive failure to recognize nouns or to recognize common objects (cat, book, glass of milk), while other cognitive abilities are unchanged. Eventually the speech becomes difficult to understand as the Person with Dementia can no longer generate the key words in sentences. Difficulty recognizing common objects and faces helps confirm this diagnosis. FTD behaviors will not be exhibited until the late stages of dementia. Swallowing issues indicate death from aspiration pneumonia, sepsis, and kidney failure (renal failure).

Logopenic Variant Primary Progressive Dementia

This dementia causes the resident to have an inability to retrieve words. She will present with a slow speech pattern dotted with pauses for significant word-finding problems. The ability to understand long and complex sentences is lost and eventually mutism is present. Reading and writing abilities continue to function

NOTES

a bit longer, but eventually decline as well. Neuroimaging demonstrates a loss of blood volume, blood flow, and neural activity in the left Temporal and Parietal Lobes. Swallowing again becomes an issue in the late stages and death occurs from aspiration pneumonia, sepsis, and kidney failure (renal failure). This variation of FTD may be closely related to Alzheimer's pathology.

Challenges

- Poor family involvement due to the loss of emotion from the person with dementia, which may lead to divorce before the dementia diagnosis is made
- Younger age of the Person with Dementia causes increased stress for family and professional caregivers.
- Rapid decline is difficult for caregivers.
- Lack of facial and vocal affect may frighten caregivers.
- Lack of emotion may frighten caregivers.

Parkinson's Disease Dementia (PDD)
Named for Dr. James Parkinson

Area(s) of the Brain

This dementia begins in the basal ganglia in the central part of the brain and then spreads into the rest of the brain. Memory functions, the ability to pay attention, make sound judgments, and demonstrate executive functioning become impaired. It is theorized that there is a strong connection between the Lewy Bodies protein alpha-synuclein, Parkinson's Disease, and Parkinson's Disease Dementia.

Complicating the disease research is the presence of tau neurofibrillary tangles and APOE protein plaques found in Alzheimer's Dementia. Visual hallucinations similar to Lewy Bodies Dementia may be experienced, delusions that have a paranoid slant, muffled or soft speech, difficulty interpreting visual information, depression, irritability, anxiety, and sleep disturbances including REM Sleep Behavior Disorder (kicking and punching in sleep) are also present.

LBD and PDD are now considered "first cousins" and caregivers should

Parkinson's Disease Brain

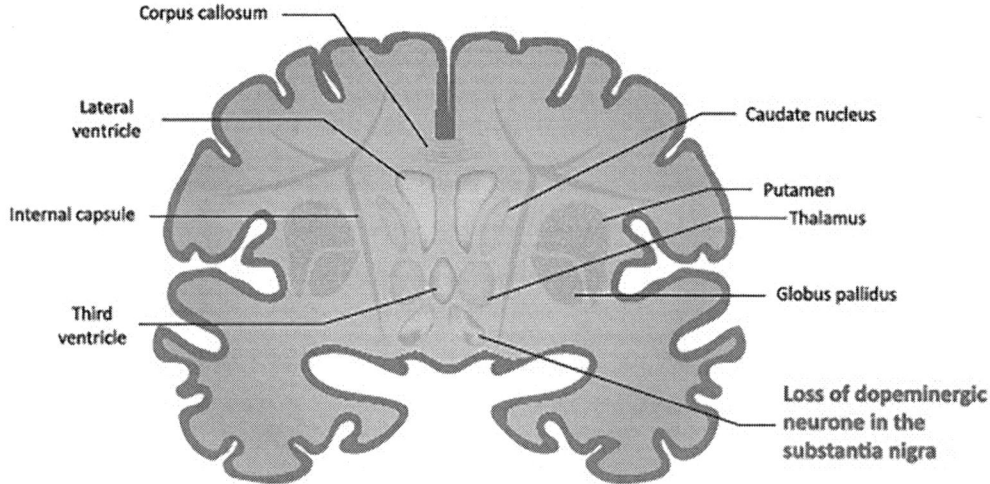

anticipate if the person has LBD, the PDD will join and vice versa, causing a form of Mixed Dementia. *(NOTE:* Hallucinations and delusions in PDD are thought more likely to be related to medication than the disease.

Falls
- Common falls are distinctly different from other dementias. People with Parkinson's Disease Dementia (PDD) stiffen and fall forward, landing on their faces or stiffen and fall backwards, cracking the crown of the skull on impact.
- The falls are frequently due to a sudden loss of consciousness.
- Parkinson's Disease Dementia falls are very similar to Lewy Bodies falls.

Order of Progression
- Being diagnosed late in life increases the likelihood that Parkinson's Disease will become Parkinson's Disease Dementia.

Anticipated Behaviors
- Slowed movements
- Muscle stiffness
- Tremor, shuffling while walking
- Masked face
- Paranoid and delusional belief
- The onset of cognitive decline
- Changes in mood and behavior begin

Challenges
- Caregiver death due to the stress of care, falls, choking

Wernicke-Korsakoff's Syndrome
Named for Dr. Carl Wernicke and Dr. Sergei Korsakoff

Area(s) of the Brain

There are multiple variations of this dementia. Wernicke Encephalopathy is recognized by features such as changes in vision and eye functioning and leg tremors. Other features include a decrease in mental alertness and an increase in confusion. This is usually the result of long-term alcoholism causing a thiamine (vitamin B-1) deficiency, although it can also be caused by cancer, severe intestinal problems, and malnutrition. Immediate treatment with hospitalization is required to monitor the intake of thiamine.

Clinical features include jerky eye movements, droopy upper eyelids, double vision, an altered mental status, poor balance, and difficulty walking. These should be documented for the physician. Persons with this dementia often appear malnourished and underweight. She frequently will have low blood pressure, a low body temperature, and new memory issues. This person may appear to be drunk even when sober. This can occur with the daily drinker or the binge drinker.

If left untreated, Wernicke Syndrome progresses to Korsakoff Syndrome. This dementia is marked by memory loss and challenges to perform the ADLs and the IADLs. She will experience more and more difficulty learning new information, as damage continues in the medial temporal lobe.

This area of the temporal lobes contains the hippocampus and limbic systems, so she will be unable to learn new information as these areas are severely damaged. Instead, she will begin to demonstrate a behavior called confabulation.

Many caregivers may misinterpret confabulation with lying, but it is not. Rather it is a unique fallback position the brain appears to use. When she cannot find the correct information because of brain damage, her brain will try to fill in

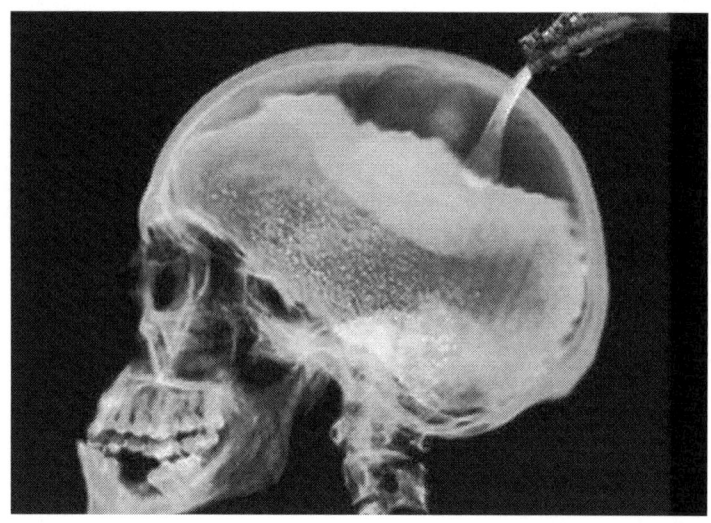

the missing gap of information with something similar.

The Thanksgiving party gets related as the Fourth of July party. She will be unaware she is confabulating and may become defensive if challenged about the facts. Her behaviors may become agitated, aggressive, impulsive, or she may withdraw from others in the community.

Death is caused by dementia complications, lung infections (pneumonia followed by sepsis -- blood poisoning from overwhelming infection, which leads to kidney failure).

Falls
• This person may fall in any direction depending upon how long she abused alcohol and what other medical conditions are present.

Order of Progression
- Damage to the amygdala, mild frontal lobe atrophy, moderately severe damage to the medial temporal lobe and atrophy.

Anticipated Behavior
- Among dementias, this group has the highest rate (28 percent) of reported scatological behavior, primarily coprophagia (eating one's own feces)
- Some people may become impulsive and grab or snatch at times.

Challenges
- Due to history of addiction and drinking related behaviors, family involvement may be sporadic.

Dementias of the Huntington's Type (HD)
Named for Dr. George Huntington
Domains:
• Huntington's Dementia • Juvenile Huntington's Disease • Huntington's Chorea

Area(s) of the Brain

The mutation of a normal gene causes the degeneration and death of the nerve cells in the basal ganglia. This is the area of the brain that coordinates movement, and the genetic mutation is passed from parent to child. The child has a fifty percent chance of having the gene.

In the middle stages of the disease, she will begin to have challenges with speaking and with swallowing. A speech therapist should be ordered by the physician to do a swallow study test. These tests will continue until death.

Walking will be very difficult, and if she develops Chorea, her jerking limbs will make it especially difficult to walk safely. Nonetheless, she will continue to attempt to walk. The jerking movement in her limbs will also make performing or assisting her with her ADLs very challenging.

As her memory becomes more damaged, she may have obsessive behaviors or fixations on items. Concentrating and staying on task are becoming more difficult for her to do, and she may become verbally agitated.

Many of the dementias are very similar by the end stage of the disease due to the overall or global loss of brain tissue or damage. Likewise, persons with Huntington's Dementia require total care and are an especially high risk for choking.

Symptoms of the disease typically begin between the ages of 30 and 50, with life expectancy after the onset of symptoms estimated at 10 to 15 years. With this inherited disease, a child is typically not tested until the age of 18, unless she is showing symptoms.

NOTES

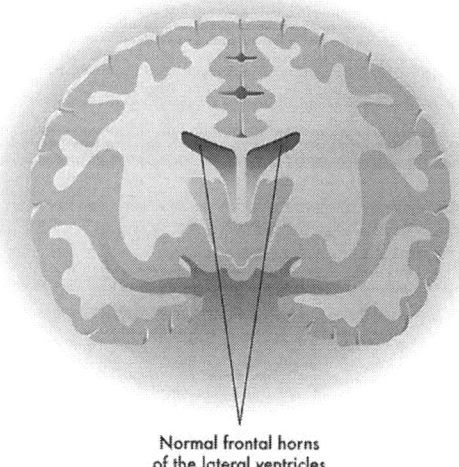
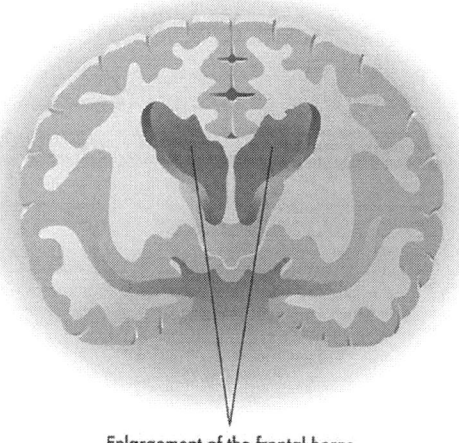

Normal brain section — Normal frontal horns of the lateral ventricles

Huntington's disease — Enlargement of the frontal horns of the lateral ventricles

Falls
- This dementia causes multiple variations of falls due to the movement disorder inherent in this form.

Order of Progression
- This group has the highest suicide rate of any of the dementias. This is thought to be due to the genetics of this disease.
- Early symptoms begin with difficulty learning new things, affecting short-term memory. She will begin having difficulty making daily decisions. She will display mood swings and involuntary movements, or twitching will begin affecting her balance and coordination. Falls and stumbles will begin.

Anticipated Behavior
- Abnormal and jerking body movements (Chorea)
- Slow bodily movement
- Increased muscle activity
- Fidgeting
- Declining cognitive skills
- Depression
- Irritability
- Anxiety
- Some patients may progress to exhibiting psychotic behaviors.

Challenges
- This is a genetic disorder inherited from a parent that affects a person's ability to think, feel, and move.
- Communication, walking, mood changes, poor decision-making skills, memory loss, and swallowing mark the progression of the disease.
- This group has the highest suicide rate of any of the dementias.

Chronic Traumatic Encephalopathy (CTE)
Named for causation and type of damage
(commonly called football or sport dementia)

Early Onset CTE
- Mood: depression, irritability, hopelessness
- Behavior: impulsivity, explosivity, aggression
- Cognitive: memory impairment, executive dysfunction, dementia
- Motor: Parkinsonism, ataxia (lack of voluntary coordination of muscle movements, including gait abnormality, eye movement abnormality, and changes in speech), dysarthria (slurred speech)
- Note: Early Onset CTE cases have a higher prevalence of motor dysfunction and are especially sensitive to alcohol

Late Onset CTE
- Mood: depression, irritability, hopelessness
- Behavior: impulsivity, explosivity, aggression
- Cognitive: memory impairment, executive dysfunction, dementia
- Motor: Parkinsonism, ataxia (lack of voluntary coordination of muscle movements –gait abnormality, eye movement abnormality, and changes in speech), dysarthria (slurred speech)

There is a recognized Mixed CTE in both forms which includes features of more than one domain.

Areas of the Brain

Repeated blows or strikes to the head resulting in a shearing effect in the frontal lobes and temporal lobes from striking against the interior frontal bone. The occipital lobes are damaged by striking the rear of the cranium and the brain stem is twisted by strikes from the side.

Damage includes significant atrophy of the cerebral hemispheres, medial temporal lobe, thalamus, mammillary bodies, and the brain stem. Testing for CTE via spinal fluid indicates extremely high numbers of tau proteins.

Falls

- There is not enough research yet to determine specific fall markers.
- The athleticism of these persons combined with the motor damage to the brain makes each case unique.

BONUS MATERIAL:
Some Behaviors in Dementia

Dementia-Specific Behavior

- Physically or verbally aggressive – Vascular
- Physically aggressive (especially with alcohol) - CTE
- Hallucination (a person sees, hears, or smells something that is not there) – Alzheimer's, Lewy Body, Parkinson's, Vascular
- Delusion (a person has a belief that is not real) – Alzheimer's, Lewy Body, Vascular
- Bathing or other ADL Challenges – Any dementia
- Sundowning – Any dementia
- Physical/Personal Space Violation, lack of empathy, early loss of language possibly leading to agitation, public masturbation – FTD
- Paranoia, persecutory, suspicious – Any dementia
- Anxiety – Vascular, FTD, Parkinson's
- Generalized Anxiety Disorder - 38-72 % of all dementias
- Coprophagia - eating feces – WKD
- Odd speech or word use – Communication FTDs

Anxiety or Pain Behaviors
- Restlessness, easily fatigued, difficulty concentrating, picking, scratching, rocking, pilling, spitting, yelling, grabbing, calling out, anxious body movement, physical or verbal agitation, short tempered, change in eating habits, gritting or grinding teeth, wringing hands, biting, or chewing nails

Also
- Hitting, kicking, pinching, facial grimaces, frowning, furrowed brow, sad expression, breathing differently, being very still or very agitated, frightened, closed eyes or rapidly blinking, sighing, moaning, groaning, chanting, tense body posture, guarding, restlessness, gait, or mobility changes, change in routine, appetite change, increased confusion

Scatological Behaviors
- Pica - eating substances with no nutritional value
- Coprophagia - eating feces - WKD
- Scatolia - smearing feces, (usually to get the hand clean)
- Urinating - corners, trash cans, plants (it's usually a guy thing)
- Defecating in strange areas (usually can't find a bathroom)

Depressive Behaviors
- Angry, annoyed, agitated, aggressive, withdrawn, tearful,
- Change in appetite, change in sleep, irritable
- Sudden explosions of behavior followed by no recognition that the behavior occurred

Self-Soothing Behaviors
- Humming, singing, talking, rocking or repetitive movements, breathing slowly, pilling, folding, following, playing, baby dolls

NOTES

Sensory Changes Effect Behavior

- *Vision* — Moves from 3D to 1D, loss of peripheral vision, floor tapping, left eye vision loss (Stage Six, also called Occipital Blindness.)
- *Hearing* — Inability to translate sound, inability to track sound, difficulty hearing higher pitch voices or sounds
- *Taste and Smell* — Retains ability to taste and smell sweets
- *Touch* - pilling, rubbing, folding behaviors

Sexual Behaviors

- Change in sexual orientation behavior
- Sexual interests — increase or decrease
- Accusations of sexual infidelity — LBD
- Public nudity — FTD
- Sex talk – Viagra – porn – FTD, LBD
- Hypersexual – LBD, Vascular, FTD
- Misinterpreting environment
- Not recognizing family members
- Resident-with-resident attraction

Anosognosia — The inability to recognize you have dementia.
Caregivers Can Cause Behaviors!

Stop asking why, stop arguing, stop correcting the Person with Dementia.

Five Things to Remember

1. People with Dementia are unaware they have dementia. They do not feel they are impaired or not thinking cognitively.
   This is called anosognosia.
2. People with Dementia are demonstrating damage in the hippocampus area when they begin to repeat questions.
3. A healthy human brain weighs about three pounds. By the end of dementia, a person's brain may weigh only one pound.
4. People with Dementia do not appear physically ill until the end stages of the disease. It is not unusual for persons in stage six to suffer a spiral or twist and turn hip fracture. Broken bones indicate the brain is now too damaged to maintain the skeletal structure and the end of life is coming.
5. Everything a Person with Dementia is doing is related to the damage occurring in her brain.

Five
STAGING DEMENTIA

All dementias, except for Chronic Traumatic Encephalopathy (CTE), are staged using a global deterioration scale of seven declines marked by changes in the person's behaviors.

The CTE dementias have four domains of Mood, Behavior, Cognition, and Motor. They are currently evaluated on a four-stage tool.

Stage I in CTE presents with:

Headaches, loss of attention, difficulty concentrating, followed by short-term memory issues, depression (atypical presentation with anger, annoyance, agitation, aggressive behaviors or outbursts), aggressive tendencies, explosivity (especially with alcohol), and decreased executive function.

Stage II in CTE presents with:

Mood swings, headache, and increased depression. There is also an increased loss of executive function, heightened impulsivity, suicidal thoughts or ideations, and increasing challenges with language use and comprehension.

Stage III in CTE presents with:

Increased loss of short-term memory, continued decline and loss of executive function, increased difficulty with concentration and attention, increase in explosivity, increased depression, great mood swings, physical and verbal aggression, visuospatial challenges. Apathy is frequently noted, and a greater presentation of cognitive impairment is observed.

© 2022 Tam Cummings, Ph.D. tamcummings.com

Stage IV in CTE presents with:

Severe loss of cognitive abilities for short-term and long-term memory, a dementia diagnosis, profound loss of attention and concentration, increased paranoia and depression, visuospatial impairment, gait disruption, loss of language, explosivity, aggression, and Parkinsonian movements.

Tools for Staging Dementias:

DBAT

The other forms of dementia are staged on the Dementia Behavioral Assessment Tool (DBAT) and the FrontoTemporal Symptoms and Staging Tool. When using the DBAT, be alert to how the person's family or caregivers are reporting the behaviors. The variations are a clue to the type of dementia.

For example, in most forms of dementia, a common Stage Five behavior is to accuse caregivers or family members of theft or infidelity. But in Dementias of the Lewy Bodies Type, this is a behavior seen earlier in the disease during Stage Three.

Most presentations of dementia will help monitor the person as they progress steadily and in sequence through the behaviors and stages. In other words, they go down a slippery slope. But if the dementia is a form of Vascular Dementia, then expect behaviors to be related to where in the brain lobes the vascular activity has occurred. For example, a person with stroke activity might be aware of today's date, but not able to remember how to transfer from a sitting to a standing position because the stroke impacted that particular area of the brain.

Persons with vascular dementias will appear to stair step through the stages. This person suffers a vascular event, such as a stroke or heart attack, recovers, stabilizes or appears to, then has another event.

FTD Symptoms and Staging Tool (FTDSST)

The FTD Symptoms and Staging Tool divides this cluster of dementias into their domains and then marks an X in the box with the behavior if that particular

NOTES

behavior is associated with that form of FTD. In Stage Six of the tool there are no more X marks because, by Stage Six, all dementias are considered the same due to the amount of brain damage.

Actively Dying Assessment Tool (ADAT)

The Actively Dying Assessment Tool allows for professional and family caregivers to track and recognize the signs and stages of the final part of life. Beginning in the final months, the tool provides the expected behaviors and physiological changes occurring in people who are actively dying.

PAINAD

This tool allows the caregiver to measure the level of pain in a Person with Dementia. Because of damage to the temporal and parietal lobes, the Person with Dementia cannot alert caregivers to pain. PRN orders — also known as orders for pain medication "as needed" — are not effective due to the inability of the Person with Dementia to recognize or request pain medication. An estimated 50 percent of the behaviors displayed by a Person with Dementia are pain related, so routine evaluations for pain are necessary to provide proper care.

Cornell Scale for Depression in Dementia

This tool is valuable to demonstrate effectiveness of interventions, especially anti-depressant treatment when it is completed before the intervention and several weeks after.

Hamilton Anxiety Rating Scale (HAM-A)

This tool utilizes a list of phrases that describe certain feelings that people have. It rates the person by finding the answer that best describes the extent to which he/she experiences these feelings on a scale of 1 to 5, with 1 being Not Present and 5 being Very Severe.

The Bristol Activities of Daily Living Scale (BADLs)EP TEST

This tool allows caregivers to recognize and report the loss of abilities displayed by the Person with Dementia. It provides professionals and family caregivers with an understanding of decline in the person's abilities.

St. Louis University Mental Status (SLUMS) Examination

The SLUMS Examination is a screening test for dementia. It is an alternative to the widely used Mini-Mental State Examination (MMSE). SLUMS was designed to identify people with early dementia symptoms, also known as mild cognitive impairment (MCI).

Short Form of the Informant Questionnaire on Cognitive Decline in Elderly (Short IQCODE)

The Short IQCODE allows a family member or friend to compare what the Person with Dementia was like 10 years ago with how they are today. It provides situations where the person had to use memory or intelligence and whether this ability has improved, stayed the same, or worsened. It provides a rating scale of 1 to 5, with 1 being Much Improved and 5 being Much Worse.

The Zarit Burden Interview

The Zarit provides caregivers a means for assessing their perceptions of burden that may inadvertently affect their health, social, or general well-being.

MM Caregiver Grief Inventory - Short Form

This tool is designed to measure the grief experience of current family caregivers or persons living with progressive dementia. It provides statements that the person rates agreement with based on a scale of 1 to 5, with 1 being Strongly Disagree and 5 being Strongly Agree.

NOTES

Geriatric Depression Scale (GDS)

This tool is a self-report measure of depression in older adults. User responds in a "Yes/No" format. It is comprised of 15 items chosen for their high correlation with depressive symptoms in previous validation studies. Of the 15 items, 10 indicate the presence of depression when answered positively, while the other five are an indication of depression when answered negatively.

Brief Psychiatric Rating Scale (BPRS)

The BPRS assesses the level of 18 symptom constructs, such as hostility, suspiciousness, hallucination, and grandiosity. It is particularly useful in gauging the efficacy of treatment in persons who have moderate to severe psychoses. The rater enters a number for each symptom construct that ranges from 1 (not present) to 7 (extremely severe).

USE THE TOOLS!

The staging tools provide family members, physicians, and caregiving staff the best picture of the disease progression in a Person with Dementia. Rechecking the tools every two months will provide a map of the rate of progression of the disease and decline in the Person with Dementia. Share them with families and professionals for the best outcomes.

NOTES

Assessment Tools

Dementia Behavioral Assessment Tool (DBAT)

	STAGE 1 or NORMAL AGING
☑	**BEHAVIOR CHARACTERISTICS**
☐	No cognitive changes evident. Normal aging, normal brain function.
	STAGE 2 or EARLY STAGE or MILD COGNITIVE IMPAIRMENT (MCI)
☑	**BEHAVIOR CHARACTERISTICS**
☐	Fleeting moments of cognitive loss
☐	Recovers relatively quickly from mistakes, may correct self
☐	Misplaces familiar objects
☐	Forgets names he/she knows well
☐	No problems completing tasks or at social functions
☐	Exhibits appropriate concern over memory function
☐	Vacillates between seeking medical care and ignoring symptoms
☐	Functions effectively at work and at home
☐	Highly functional social skills
☐	Requires complete cognitive testing to determine illness
☐	Responds to cognitive therapy
☐	Scores well on orientation test
☐	Amnesia[1] beginning to be expressed
☐	May become defensive when questioned
☐	Easily irritable
☐	Easily frustrated by common tasks
	STAGE 3 or MIDDLE STAGE or BEGINNING DEMENTIA
Minimal brain tissue lost	**Stage thought to last 1-4 years**
Abilities equivalent of teenager to adulthood	
☑	**BEHAVIOR CHARACTERISTICS**
☐	Memory deficit evident in intensive interview
☐	Attempts to conceal deficits and denies any cognition difficulties
☐	Expresses concern regarding deficits (mild/moderate anxiety)
☐	Problems performing in demanding situations (work or social)
☐	Co-workers/family members beginning to be aware of increasing challenges
☐	Can get lost traveling to new areas
☐	Exhibits signs of cognition but may retain little new information
☐	Name/Word finding difficulty more frequent
☐	Challenged to remember new names
☐	May appear depressed
☐	Demonstrates high social skill level
☐	Uses humor to avoid answering questions
☐	No noticeable physical changes, but may begin stumbling or falling or sleeping excessively
☐	Beginning to skip steps in tasks

© 2022 Tam Cummings, Ph.D. tamcummings.com

Dementia Behavioral Assessment Tool (DBAT), continued

☐	Able to score well on orientation test, but not on cognition exam
☐	At times appears befuddled or confused
☐	Amnesia[1] and Aphasia[2] present - needs new information repeated
☐	Increased episodes of sudden irritability
☐	Quickly agitated and defensive of memory
☐	Sundowning may begin

LBD	Accuses caregiver of theft
	Hallucinations: (common ones) 1) children, 2) bugs, spiders, rats, snakes, 3) bad people coming to hurt or kill him/her, 4) sees caregiver having sex with others
	Rapid onset of depression, suicide risk
	Loss of facial and vocal affect may begin

STAGE 4 or MIDDLE STAGE or MODERATE DEMENTIA

Stage thought to last 1-4 years	4 ounces brain tissue loss
Abilities equivalent of adulthood to teenager	

☑	**BEHAVIOR CHARACTERISTICS**
☐	Decreased knowledge of current and recent events
☐	Memory deficits regarding personal history, may look to spouse to answer questions
☐	Decreased ability to perform serial subtractions (100-7, 93-7, 86-7, etc.)
☐	Difficulty with immediate recall – repeats statements or questions or calls without recognizing he or she has already done or asked these things multiple times
☐	Difficulty with complex tasks such as driving, finances, shopping, bathing
☐	Denial of deficits, with or without agitation or annoyance, but expect annoyance or anger
☐	Withdraws from challenging situations - refuses to complete tasks, may make excuses
☐	Increased anxiety/frustration abilities or loss of abilities
☐	Difficulty telling jokes, stories - starting to mix up stories (confabulation, not lying)
☐	Decreased facial affect (emotion on face)
☐	Increased depressive symptoms, possibly Atypical[8]: anxiety, anger, agitation, aggression
☐	May hesitate when trying to correctly identify family members or close friends
☐	Can have normal cognition for hours or days, then become quite confused
☐	May become lost in tasks, stuck on a step and unable to figure out the next step
☐	Greater language challenges, word-finding difficulty
☐	Begins to have stumbles or falls
☐	May begin to shadow caregiver
☐	Begins to have difficulty with (ADLS are lost last because humans learned these things first) ADLs[6] or (IADLS are lost first because they were learned as teenagers and young adults) IADLs[7]
☐	May begin keeping lists of family names, phone numbers, etc.
☐	Exhibits greater desire for sweet foods
☐	May score well on orientation test, dementia evident on cognition exam
☐	Amnesia[1], Aphasia[2], Agnosia[3], and Anosognosia[4] present, some paranoia present
Nursing:	Coordination beginning to be impaired Family Caregiver's Health beginning to be impacted by the care Family Caregiver is now performing IADLs and some ADLs

© 2022 Tam Cummings, Ph.D. tamcummings.com

Dementia Behavioral Assessment Tool (DBAT), continued

	Family Caregiver is now at risk for Compassion Fatigue or Secondary Traumatic Stress Disorder Person With Dementia is not safe to drive Person With Dementia is becoming a risk to self for care (medications, foods, driving, finances, exploitation, etc.)
	**EARLY STAGE 5 or LATE STAGE or MODERATELY SEVERE DEMENTIA**
Stage thought to last 1-3 years	1/2 to 1 pound of brain tissue loss
	Abilities equivalent of 12 - 8 year old – should be in Memory Care or a Skilled Facility
☑	**BEHAVIOR CHARACTERISTICS**
☐	Disorientation to time (date, day of week, season, etc.) or place
☐	Immediate memory relatively intact - knows self and family
☐	May need assistance choosing and layering clothing, but denies need for IADL/ADL
☐	May crave sweets over other foods
☐	Begins to have falls
☐	Hunting and gathering stage, wanders from room to room collecting items
☐	Urinary incontinence begins - monthly to weekly to daily
☐	Wears clothing appropriately (hearing aid, glasses, carries purse)
☐	*Feeds self (may need meal set-up)
☐	Sleep disturbances, excessive sleeping or napping
☐	Can score well on an orientation test, but not a cognition test
☐	Wanders looking for a way out (purposeful wandering/ Sundowning)
☐	Follows simple instructions for ADLs, verbal cues needed for tasks
☐	Unexplained tearfulness or extreme laughter (pseudo bulbar – see doctor ASAP)
☐	Catastrophic reactions - may be easily annoyed, agitated, verbally or physically aggressive if pushed to perform ADL or IADL or answer questions
☐	Hallucinations, accusatory behavior, excessive sleeping - report to doctor
☐	Amnesia[1], Aphasia[2], Agnosia[3], and Anosognosia[4,] and Apraxia[5] evident to outsiders
☐	May make comments about death
Nursing:	Vital signs should be stable
	Begin recording monthly body temperature and weight
	Begin PAINAD monitoring Family Caregiver grieving at Post Death Grief Levels Family Caregiver's health remains at risk
	**MIDDLE LATE STAGE 5 or LATE STAGE or MODERATELY SEVERE DEMENTIA**
	Abilities equivalent of 8 - 4 year old – Should be in Memory Care or Skilled Care
	BEHAVIOR CHARACTERISTICS
☐	May begin having chronic Urinary Tract Infections (UTIs)
☐	Appears severely depressed with increased loss of facial affect
☐	Increased fall risks, may not recognize severity of the fall especially to the head
☐	Coordinated movement/function beginning to be affected Can't start the social skill but response to the cue

© 2022 Tam Cummings, Ph.D. tamcummings.com

Dementia Behavioral Assessment Tool (DBAT), continued

	LATE STAGE 5 or LATE STAGE or MODERATELY SEVERE DEMENTIA continued
☐	Begins to be lost in current time
☐	Difficulty recognizing self in a mirror
☐	Challenged to recall family members, may confuse daughter with mother, etc
	Accuses family members, caregivers of theft, infidelity, lying, increased paranoia possible
☐	Automatic "yes/no" speech functions, but without understanding
☐	May begin using curse words as temporal lobes become damaged
☐	Changes in visual perception increasing, bumps into objects, peripheral vision damaged
☐	Difficulty interpreting background noise
☐	Challenged to perform rehab for injuries, may appear stubborn to therapist/family
☐	Cannot give accurate information, verbal skills damaged
☐	Caregivers may confuse behavior for purposeful active - lying, etc.
☐	Physical Appearance beginning to be affected
☐	Pilling or rubbing hand motions common, may enjoy folding items
Nursing:	Hyperoral behavior may begin
	UTIs require culture and sensitivity (C&S) orders
	Continue monthly body, temperature, and weight checks
	Sleep disturbance beginning

	STAGE 6 or LATE STAGE or SEVERE DEMENTIA
Stage thought to last 1-3 years	**1 to 1 1/2 pounds of brain tissue loss**
Abilities equivalent of 4 - 2 year old	
☑	**BEHAVIOR CHARACTERISTICS**
☐	Unable to recall most recent events
☐	Repetitiveness in motion or speech or memory
☐	May be in constant motion, wanders/walks for hours
☐	Removes/won't wear clothing appropriately
☐	Disregards eyeglasses, dentures, hearing aids (Agnosia[3]) - may throw them away
☐	Refuses to change clothing, unable to complete IADLs and a few ADLs
☐	*Feeds self with set-up, cues and assistance
☐	Bowel incontinence begins
☐	Sleep disturbances - may increase sleep, may require little sleep
☐	Catastrophic reactions may occur - great resistance to care giving, bathing
☐	Purposeless wandering/Sun-downing (wandering without an agenda)
☐	Cannot complete a two-stage command, such as pick up a piece of paper and fold it
☐	Apraxia[5] advanced, gait altered (small shuffling steps)
☐	Weight loss beginning, may lose 1/3 or more of body weight
☐	Difficult to engage with caregiver, challenged to initiate conversation
☐	Disheveled appearance
☐	Fall risk continues to increase until wheelchair bound, risk for fractured bones increases
☐	Difficult to perform rehab for injuries
☐	Almost total loss of facial affect

© 2022 Tam Cummings, Ph.D. tamcummings.com

Dementia Behavioral Assessment Tool (DBAT), continued

	May suddenly use complete sentence, then only words or sounds
	Ability to taste sweets drives appetite
	**Extensive brain tissue loss and/or damage**
Nurses Care plan:	Begins weight loss of 1/3 to 1/2 body weight
	Add high calorie snacks and finger foods
	Spiral fracture of hip (6x more likely to break bones)
	Full set vitals and weight monthly
	Occipital blindness - left eye doesn't function
	Speech Therapist evaluation ordered when pocketing, choking, swallowing issues noted with food or liquid
	Falls now directly linked to pre-motor cortex damage
	Hyperoral possibility
	Routine performance of Braden Scale for Predicting Pressure Sore Risk
	Monthly PAINAD review - pulse increases with pain Battle's Sign ear bruising
	Monitor clothing for warmth as body temperature drops

STAGE 7 or LATE STAGE or VERY SEVERE DEMENTIA

Stage thought to last 1-2 years	1 1/2 - 2 pounds of brain tissue loss

Abilities equivalent of 2 year old to infant

☑	**BEHAVIOR CHARACTERISTICS**
☐	Frequently no speech at all - mostly grunting or word sounds
☐	*Cannot feed self --- chipmunking or holding food in cheeks, high risk for choking
☐	Unable to sit up independently, unable to hold head up
☐	Loss of basic psychomotor skills (unable to walk w/o assistance)
☐	Hyperoral (may put everything in mouth)
☐	Displays great muscular flexation, hands curl, arms and legs pull up
☐	Extreme risk for skin breakdown leading to wounds (Braden Scale*)
☐	Spends majority of day asleep or semi-alert, but understands tone of caregiver
☐	Extreme weight loss
☐	Loss of ability to smile -- indicates death is near
☐	Total care required
Nursing	PAINAD review monthly
	Braden Scale - weekly then daily as skin integrity is threatened

ACTIVELY DYING ASSESSMENT TOOL (ADAT)
The Final Months

	Significant change in health Should be stable and isn't
	Clear and vivid dreams are reported
	Talks about missing a loved one
	Adult Failure to Thrive diagnosis may be made
	Withdraw from social/family activities

© 2022 Tam Cummings, Ph.D. tamcummings.com

Dementia Behavioral Assessment Tool (DBAT), continued

	The Final Weeks - Skin breakdown risk increases. Especially buttocks, hips, and heels.
	Less eye contact, more withdrawn
	Looking and/or reaching beyond and above
	Reports seeing/talking to favorite persons
	Increased risk of falling
	Less interest in food or drink
	Conversations with people not there
	Reports people are telling him/her to "Come on"
	May report strange feelings in limbs
	Tires easily
	Voice Weakens easily
	The Final Days
	May have fever followed by sweats
	May speak to family members who have already died

	Even less interest in food or drink
	General restlessness displayed
	Leg tremors may occur
	Pulse and breathing start to slow
	Kidney and liver function start to slow
	Circulation slowing - reposition every 2 hours
	May begin breathing through mouth
	Respiration will pick up and slow down repeatedly
	May Have Sudden Alert Time and Ravenous Hunger
	The Final Hours
	Fever may come and go
	Overall calmness, but may pick at covers or PJ's
	May not respond to sound or speech
	Eyes may not follow movement around room
	Exhibits "doll's eyes"
	Trembling/twitching in limbs/sometimes violent
	Gurgling in throat ("Death Rattle")
	Bruising from blood clotting system failing
	Semi-comatose appearance
	Breathing through mouth
	Kidney function very slow, urine becomes dark
	Mottling - blue/purple color in feet or hands
	Pressure wounds may open (bed sores) in hours
	Heart rate slows
	Respiration slows to <14 breaths per minute and may rise and fall for hours
	Odor may be present
	Apnea begins (stops breathing between breaths)

© 2022 Tam Cummings, Ph.D. tamcummings.com

Dementia Behavioral Assessment Tool (DBAT), continued

	Cheyne-Stokes (Chain-Stokes) breathing Death is now minutes or hours away
	Final Breath
	May make a "pa" sound or spittle/foam at mouth
	Death
	Body appears to shrink almost immediately
	Body becomes pale, cool, and gray
	Eyes and mouth typically remain open
	Eyes flatten from loss of blood pressure
	Body may have slight settling movement
	Body may release urine or stool

Amnesia[1] - the inability to use or retain short-term or long-term memory

Aphasia[2] - the inability to use or understand language

Agnosia[3] - the inability to use or recognize common objects or people

Anosognosia[4] - the inability to recognize impaired function (not denial) in memory, general thinking skills, emotions and body functions

Apraxia[5] - the inability to use coordinated and purposeful muscle movement

ADLs[6] - Katz's Index of Independence in Activities of Daily Living - bathing, dressing, toileting, transferring, continence and feeding

IADLs[7] - Lawton-Brody Instrumental Activities of Daily Living - the ability to use a telephone, shopping, food preparation, housekeeping, laundry, mode of transportation, responsibility for own medication

Atypical Depression[8] - is a form of depression more commonly seen in dementia. Person appear aggressive - either verbally or physically or both, angry, anxious, agitated and/or annoyed

Braden Scale for Predicting Pressure Sore Risk* - developed to foster early identification of patients at risk for forming pressure sores. The scale is composed of six subscales that reflect sensory perception, skin moisture, activity, mobility, friction and shear, and nutritional status

*Food preparation moves from regular to mechanically chopped to finger foods to pureed. Your doctor will write an order for a speech therapist to evaluate your lovedone's ability to chew and swallow foods and liquids

The FrontoTemporal Dementia Symptoms and Staging Tool — FTD-SST

FrontoTemporal Dementia Stages & Symptoms	Behavioral Personality FTD		Communication & Language FTD			Motor & Movement Disorder FTD			
	bvFTD — Behavioral Variant FTD**	Pick's Disease**	PPA — Primary Progressive Aphasia	Semantic Dementia**	Logopengic Variant PSP**	ProSupra Nuclear Palsy PSP**	Corticobasal Ganglionic Degeneration	FTD with Motor Neuron Disease	ALS with Dementia

FrontoTemporal Dementia (FTD) is named because it primarily affects the frontal and temporal lobes. It is the most common dementia between the ages of 40-60. Sometimes referred to as Fronto-Temporal Lobar Degeneration, the term FTLD is the post mortem name.

Stage 1 — Normal Aging

Stage 2 — Typical First Signs and Early Depression Symptoms*

Symptom									
Alterations in alertness									
Apathy									
Slow withdrawal of emotional responses									
Agitation									
Bursts of anger									
* Signs of disinterest									
* Apathy not related to being sad									
* Little insight into being sad									
* No self awareness of changes in mood									
* Increased irritability									
* Poor concentration									
* Lack of attention during interaction									
* Sadness or negative mood									
* Poor appetite or increased over eating									
* Insomnia or hypersomnia									
*** If sleeping more than 14 hours/day, increased risk for infections and atrophied muscles									

Stage 3 — Early Stage Symptoms

Symptom									
Sudden interest in drinking	x								
Gradual loss of empathic response	x	x							
Decreased insight into behavior	x	x							
Shoplifting	x	x							
Increase in weight — 40lbs in 6 months	x	x							
Self-centered behavior	x	x							

© 2022 Tam Cummings, Ph.D. tamcummings.com

The FrontoTemporal Dementia Symptoms and Staging Tool — FTD-SST, continued

FrontoTemporal Dementia Stages & Symptoms	Behavioral Personality FTD		Communication & Language FTD			Motor & Movement Disorder FTD			
FrontoTemporal Dementia (FTD) is named because it primarily affects the frontal and temporal lobes. It is the most common dementia between the ages of 40-60. Sometimes referred to as Fronto-Temporal Lobar Degeneration, the term FTLD is the post mortem name.	bvFTD — Behavioral Variant FTD**	Pick's Disease**	PPA — Primary Progressive Aphasia	Semantic Dementia**	Logopengic Variant PSP**	ProSupra Nuclear Palsy PSP**	Corticobasal Ganglionic Degeneration	FTD with Motor Neuron Disease	ALS with Dementia
Stage 3 — Early Stage Symptoms									
Uncaring behavior	x	x							
Withdrawal from people and activities	x	x							
Increase in spontaneous behavior, such as inappropriate friendliness, speaking candidly, revealing personal information to strangers, becoming angry during routine tasks at job or at home, may appear restless or irritable	x	x	x						
Unusual eating habits, such as food fixation (eating too much of a specific food), great craving for sweets, sucking and chewing on objects (pens, combs, spoons, etc.), hyper oral, shovel food	x	x	x						
Ignores social etiquette and boundaries, such as getting too close when speaking to others, tendency to hug, touch, talk in inappropriate or intimate ways (new behaviors for this person)	x	x	x						
Displays poor judgment	x	x	x	x					
Loss of facial empathy — masked face	x	x				x			
Decreased interest in spouse, children, family	x	x	x	x	x	x	x	x	x
Very mild short-term memory loss	x	x	x	x	x	x	x	x	x
Personal hygiene changes	x	x	x	x	x	x	x	x	x
Math skills good	x	x	x	x	x	x	x	x	x
Visual ability good	x	x	x	x	x			x	x
Mild word-finding difficulty (anomia)			x	x	x				

© 2022 Tam Cummings, Ph.D. tamcummings.com

The FrontoTemporal Dementia Symptoms and Staging Tool — FTD-SST, continued

FrontoTemporal Dementia Stages & Symptoms	Behavioral Personality FTD — bvFTD — Behavioral Variant FTD**	Behavioral Personality FTD — Pick's Disease**	Communication & Language FTD — PPA — Primary Progressive Aphasia	Communication & Language FTD — Semantic Dementia**	Communication & Language FTD — Logopenic Variant PSP**	Motor & Movement Disorder FTD — ProSupra Nuclear Palsy PSP**	Motor & Movement Disorder FTD — Corticobasal Ganglionic Degeneration	Motor & Movement Disorder FTD — FTD with Motor Neuron Disease	Motor & Movement Disorder FTD — ALS with Dementia
FrontoTemporal Dementia (FTD) is named because it primarily affects the frontal and temporal lobes. It is the most comon dementia between the ages of 40-60. Sometimes referred to as Fronto-Temporal Lobar Degeneration, the term FTLD is the post mortem name.									
Apathetic appearance in whole body			x	x	x			x	
Difficulty moving whole body or parts of body						x	x	x	x
Struggles to form words (dysarthia)			x	x	x	x			
Trembling limbs						x			
Balance problems						x			
Tipsy walking gait						x			
Exhibits doll's eyes — an inability to coordinate eye movements or aim the eye quickly up and down						x			
Acalculia — difficulty with math						x	x		
Stiff muscles in motion or when still							x		
Clumsy with one side of body (asymmetrical decline)							x		
Stiffness in one arm, followed by stiffness in one leg (paratonia)							x		
Alien hand movements — hand pushes away other objects or other hand							x		
Magnetic hand — hand seems drawn to other hand or other people's hands							x		
Fasciculations (muscle twitches or flutters)								x	
Muscle jerks								x	
Muscle cramps								x	
Loss of muscle tone								x	x

© 2022 Tam Cummings, Ph.D. tamcummings.com

The FrontoTemporal Dementia Symptoms and Staging Tool — FTD-SST, continued

FrontoTemporal Dementia Stages & Symptoms	Behavioral Personality FTD		Communication & Language FTD			Motor & Movement Disorder FTD			
	bvFTD — Behavioral Variant FTD**	Pick's Disease**	PPA — Primary Progressive Aphasia	Semantic Dementia**	Logopenic Variant PSP**	ProSupra Nuclear Palsy PSP**	Corticobasal Ganglionic Degeneration	FTD with Motor Neuron Disease	ALS with Dementia
FrontoTemporal Dementia (FTD) is named because it primarily affects the frontal and temporal lobes. It is the most common dementia between the ages of 40-60. Sometimes referred to as Fronto-Temporal Lobar Degeneration, the term FTLD is the post mortem name.									
Increase in falls and falls with injury						x	x	x	x
Difficulty doing skilled hand movements with one or both hands or arms (apraxia), which may result in difficulty buttoning shirt, turning book pages, shaving, applying makeup, eating, writing, etc.						x	x	x	x
Stage 4 — Early Middle Stage									
Judgement	x	x							
Rational thought	x	x							
Personality changes	x	x							
Impulse control	x	x							
Little concern about losses	x	x							
Rapid Eye Movement Disorder (REMD) — sleep disturbances	x	x							
Thrashing, kicking, punching, striking out while sleeping	x	x							
Can read and write accurately	x	x		x	x				
Loss or changes in executive function, such as time management, attention management, switch focus, plan and problem solve, integrate past experience with present	x	x					x		
Difficulty expressing words — nonfluent asphasia			x						
Incorrect grammar			x	x					

© 2022 Tam Cummings, Ph.D. tamcummings.com

The FrontoTemporal Dementia Symptoms and Staging Tool — FTD-SST, continued

FrontoTemporal Dementia Stages & Symptoms	Behavioral Personality FTD — bvFTD — Behavioral Variant FTD**	Pick's Disease**	Communication & Language FTD — PPA — Primary Progressive Aphasia	Semantic Dementia**	Logopenic Variant PSP**	Motor & Movement Disorder FTD — ProSupra Nuclear Palsy PSP**	Corticobasal Ganglionic Degeneration	FTD with Motor Neuron Disease	ALS with Dementia
FrontoTemporal Dementia (FTD) is named because it primarily affects the frontal and temporal lobes. It is the most common dementia between the ages of 40-60. Sometimes referred to as Fronto-Temporal Lobar Degeneration, the term FTLD is the post mortem name.									
Difficulty naming objects or recognizing familiar words or faces			x	x					
Performs ADLs			x	x	x				
Slow response to conversation			x	x	x				
Slow, weak, slurred, breathy, nasal speech (dysarthia)			x					x	
Speaks at a normal rate — fluent aphasia, but may be difficult to understand				x					
Difficulty understanding speech of others				x					
Expresses appropriate emotions				x					
Slow rate of speech					x				
Can repeat short, single words					x				
Outbursts of laughing or crying						x			
Akinesia — absence or slowed movement						x	x		
Bradykinesia — lack of spontaneous movement							x		
Shortness of breath due to weak muscles								x	x
Stage 5 — Late Middle Stage									
Loss of insight									
Repetition of behaviors									
Memory problems	x	x							
Severe cognitive deficits	x	x							
Language skills function late	x	x							

© 2022 Tam Cummings, Ph.D. tamcummings.com

The FrontoTemporal Dementia Symptoms and Staging Tool — FTD-SST, continued

FrontoTemporal Dementia Stages & Symptoms	Behavioral Personality FTD — bvFTD — Behavioral Variant FTD**	Pick's Disease**	Communication & Language FTD — PPA — Primary Progressive Aphasia	Semantic Dementia**	Logopenic Variant PSP**	Motor & Movement Disorder FTD — ProSupra Nuclear Palsy PSP**	Corticobasal Ganglionic Degeneration	FTD with Motor Neuron Disease	ALS with Dementia
FrontoTemporal Dementia (FTD) is named because it primarily affects the frontal and temporal lobes. It is the most common dementia between the ages of 40-60. Sometimes referred to as Fronto-Temporal Lobar Degeneration, the term FTLD is the post mortem name.									
Visuospatial skills still functional	x	x							
Great loss of affect — mask face	x	x	x	x	x	x	x	x	x
Increased sleep for day and night	x	x	x	x	x	x	x	x	x
Difficulty swallowing	x	x	x	x	x	x	x	x	x
Urinary incontinence	x	x	x	x	x	x	x	x	x
Severe loss of empathy	x	x	x	x	x	x	x	x	x
Difficulty adjusting mood to situation	x	x				x	x	x	
Emotional ups and downs	x	x					x		
Hesitance and slowed speech			x	x	x	x	x		
Loss of language fluidity			x	x	x				
Mutism			x	x	x				
Decreased motor movement skills						x	x	x	x
Short-term memory loss						x	x	x	x
Muscle atrophy						x	x	x	x
Struggles to form words (dysarthia)						x	x		
Abnormal posturing or frozen movements							x	x	
Unaware of one side of body							x		
Inability to balance — sitting or walking							x		
Reflexes are overactive								x	
Stage 6 — Late Stage Symptoms									
Short-term/long-term memory affected									
May stay in constant motion, walks or moves for hours									

© 2022 Tam Cummings, Ph.D. tamcummings.com

The FrontoTemporal Dementia Symptoms and Staging Tool — FTD-SST, continued

FrontoTemporal Dementia Stages & Symptoms	Behavioral Personality FTD		Communication & Language FTD			Motor & Movement Disorder FTD			
	bvFTD — Behavioral Variant FTD**	Pick's Disease**	PPA — Primary Progressive Aphasia	Semantic Dementia**	Logopenic Variant PSP**	ProSupra Nuclear Palsy PSP**	Corticobasal Ganglionic Degeneration	FTD with Motor Neuron Disease	ALS with Dementia
Disheveled appearance									
Beginning of severe weight loss									
Bowel incontinence begins									
Can feed self at times									
Great loss of language/mutism									
Difficult to engage									
Appears lost in own world									
Loss of total facial affect — masked									
Gait is greatly affected									
Combative or aggressive behavior									
Difficult to rehab									
Disregards eyeglasses, hearing aids, dentures									
Stage 7 — End Stage Symptoms									
Unable to sit erect									
Unable to walk									
Speech is lost									
Unable to hold head erect									
Extreme risk for falls									
Extreme risk for skin breakdown									
Semi-alert or asleep most of day									
Loss of ability to chew and swallow food properly									

FrontoTemporal Dementia (FTD) is named because it primarily affects the frontal and temporal lobes. It is the most common dementia between the ages of 40-60. Sometimes referred to as Fronto-Temporal Lobar Degeneration, the term FTLD is the post mortem name.

© 2022 Tam Cummings, Ph.D. tamcummings.com

The FrontoTemporal Dementia Symptoms and Staging Tool — FTD-SST, continued

FrontoTemporal Dementia Stages & Symptoms	Behavioral Personality FTD		Communication & Language FTD			Motor & Movement Disorder FTD			
FrontoTemporal Dementia (FTD) is named because it primarily affects the frontal and temporal lobes. It is the most common dementia between the ages of 40-60. Sometimes referred to as Fronto-Temporal Lobar Degeneration, the term FTLD is the post mortem name.	bvFTD — Behavioral Variant FTD**	Pick's Disease**	PPA — Primary Progressive Aphasia	Semantic Dementia**	Logopenic Variant PSP**	ProSupra Nuclear Palsy PSP**	Corticobasal Ganglionic Degeneration	FTD with Motor Neuron Disease	ALS with Dementia
Disinterest in food or drink									
Extreme weight loss									
Total care for all ADLs									
Loss of ability to smile — indicative that death is near									
** Some of the FTDs are recognized as tauopathy disease. Tau is a protein found in the brain's cellular structure. Once tau begins to fold incorrectly in the cells, it disrupts and destroys the brain's ability to function. Alzheimer's Disease is also a tauopathy. This probably h elps explain why persons with FTD eventually begin to have many of the same late symptoms as persons with Alzheimer's Disease.									

Actively Dying Assessment Tool (ADAT)

The Final Months

✓		✓	
	Significant change in health		Adult Failure to Thrive diagnosis may be made
	Clear and vivid dreams are reported		Withdraw from social/family activities
	Talks about missing a loved one		Less interest in food and drink

The Final Weeks

	Less eye contact, more withdrawn		Conversations with people not there
	Looking and/or reaching beyond and above		Reports people are telling him/her to "come on"
	Reports seeing/talking to favorite persons		May report strange feelings in limbs
	Increased risk of falling		Tires easily
	Less interest in food or drink		Voice weakens easily

Don't be afraid of silence.

The Final Days

	May have fever followed by sweats		Pulse and breathing start to slow
	Even less interest in food or drink		Kidney and liver function start to slow
	General restlessness displayed		Circulation slowing — reposition every 2 hours
	Leg tremors may occur		May begin breathing through the mouth

May have sudden alert time and ravenous hunger

Have you…

	Cried in front of your loved one		Said, "I am hurt."
	Said, "I love you."		Said, "I am lost."
	Said, "I am sad." or "I am angry."		Said, "I will miss you."
	Given your loved one permission to go.		Talked about death.

The Final Hours

	Fever may come and go		Kidney function very slow, urine becomes dark
	Overall calmness, but may pick at covers or PJs		Mottling — blue/purple color in feet and hands
	May not respond to sound or speech		Pressure wounds may open (bed sores)
	Exhibits "doll's eyes"		Respiration slows to <14 breaths per minute
	Trembling/twitching in limbs/sometimes violent		Odor may be present
	Gurgling in throat ("Death Rattle")		Apnea begins (stops breathing in between breaths)
	Semi-comatose appearance		Final breath
	Breathing through mouth		May make a "pa" sound or spittle/foam at mouth

© 2022 Tam Cummings, Ph.D. tamcummings.com

Actively Dying Assessment Tool (ADAT), continued

	Death		
✔	Body appears to shrink almost immediately	✔	Eyes flatten
	Body becomes pale, cool and gray		Body may have slight settling movement
	Eyes and mouth typically remain open		Body may release urine or stool

Grief after death, you may...

	Feel numb. Be careful driving for several months		Feel agitated and have angry outbursts
	Feel physically worse or develop colds		Momentarily forget your loved one is gone
	Feel regretful over lost time		Feel forgetful and have trouble concentrating
	Feel anger over your loss		Experience a moment of seeing her/him again
	Feel physically ill		Have dreams about your loved one
	Feel strange sensations in your body		Feel little support. Grieving takes years, not days.

© 2022 Tam Cummings, Ph.D. tamcummings.com

Use the Actively Dying Assessment Tool (ADAT) to assess Stage 7 care needs. ADAT is available online at www.tamcummings.com

FOOTNOTES

1 - Amnesia

The inability to use or retain short-term or long-term memory.

2 - Aphasia

The inability to use or understand language.

3 - Agnosia

The inability to use or recognize common objects or people.

4 - Anosognosia

The inability to recognize impaired function (not denial) in memory, general thinking skills, emotions and body functions.

5 - Apraxia

The inability to use coordinated an purposeful muscle movement.

6 - ADLs

Katz's Index of Independence in Activities of Daily Living — bathing, dressing, toileting, transferring, continence and feeding.

7 - IADLs

Lawton-Brody Instrumental Activities of Daily Living — the ability to use a telephone, shop, prepare food, perform housekeeping tasks, do laundry, utilize modes of transportation and be responsible for one's own medication needs.

8 - Atypical Depression

A form of depression more commonly seen in Persons with Dementia. The person appears aggressive — either verbally or physically or both — angry, anxious, agitated and/or annoyed.

* Food preparation moves from regular to mechanically chopped to finger foods to pureed. Your doctor will write an order for a speech therapist to evaluate your loved one's ability to chew and swallow food and liquids.

Pain Assessment in Advanced Dementia Scale (PAINAD)

Instructions: Observe the patient for five minutes before scoring his or her behaviors. Score the behaviors according to the following chart. Definitions of each item are provided on the following page. The patient can be observed under different conditions (e.g., at rest, during a pleasant activity, during caregiving, after the administration of pain medication).

Behavior	0	1	2	**Score**
Breathing Independent of vocalization	• Normal	• Occasional labored breathing • Short period of hyperventilation	• Noisy labored breathing • Long period of hyperventilation • Cheyne-Stokes respirations	
Negative vocalization	• None	• Occasional moan or groan • Low-level speech with a negative or disapproving quality	• Repeated troubled calling out • Loud moaning or groaning • Crying	
Facial expression	• Smiling or inexpressive	• Sad • Frightened • Frown	• Facial grimacing	
Body language	• Relaxed	• Tense • Distressed pacing • Fidgeting	• Rigid • Fists clenched • Knees pulled up • Pulling or pushing away • Striking out	
Consolability	• No need to console	• Distracted or reassured by voice or touch	• Unable to console, distract, or reassure	
			TOTAL SCORE	

(Warden et al., 2003)

Scoring:
The total score ranges from 0-10 points. A possible interpretation of the scores is: 1-3=mild pain; 4-6=moderate pain; 7-10=severe pain. These ranges are based on a standard 0-10 scale of pain, but have not been substantiated in the literature for this tool.

Source:
Warden V, Hurley AC, Volicer L. Development and psychometric evaluation of the Pain Assessment in Advanced Dementia (PAINAD) scale. *J Am Med Dir Assoc*. 2003;4(1):9-15.

PAINAD Item Definitions
(Warden et al., 2003)

Breathing
1. *Normal breathing* is characterized by effortless, quiet, rhythmic (smooth) respirations.
2. *Occasional labored breathing* is characterized by episodic bursts of harsh, difficult, or wearing respirations.
3. *Short period of hyperventilation* is characterized by intervals of rapid, deep breaths lasting a short period of time.
4. *Noisy labored breathing* is characterized by negative-sounding respirations on inspiration or expiration. They may be loud, gurgling, wheezing. They appear strenuous or wearing.
5. *Long period of hyperventilation* is characterized by an excessive rate and depth of respirations lasting a considerable time.
6. *Cheyne-Stokes respirations* are characterized by rhythmic waxing and waning of breathing from very deep to shallow respirations with periods of apnea (cessation of breathing).

Negative Vocalization
1. *None* is characterized by speech or vocalization that has a neutral or pleasant quality.
2. *Occasional moan or groan* is characterized by mournful or murmuring sounds, wails, or laments. Groaning is characterized by louder than usual inarticulate involuntary sounds, often abruptly beginning and ending.
3. *Low level speech with a negative or disapproving quality* is characterized by muttering, mumbling, whining, grumbling, or swearing in a low volume with a complaining, sarcastic, or caustic tone.
4. *Repeated troubled calling out* is characterized by phrases or words being used over and over in a tone that suggests anxiety, uneasiness, or distress.
5. *Loud moaning or groaning* is characterized by mournful or murmuring sounds, wails, or laments in much louder than usual volume. Loud groaning is characterized by louder than usual inarticulate involuntary sounds, often abruptly beginning and ending.
6. *Crying* is characterized by an utterance of emotion accompanied by tears. There may be sobbing or quiet weeping.

Facial Expression
1. *Smiling or inexpressive.* Smiling is characterized by upturned corners of the mouth, brightening of the eyes, and a look of pleasure or contentment. Inexpressive refers to a neutral, at ease, relaxed, or blank look.
2. *Sad* is characterized by an unhappy, lonesome, sorrowful, or dejected look. There may be tears in the eyes.
3. *Frightened* is characterized by a look of fear, alarm, or heightened anxiety. Eyes appear wide open.
4. *Frown* is characterized by a downward turn of the corners of the mouth. Increased facial wrinkling in the forehead and around the mouth may appear.
5. *Facial grimacing* is characterized by a distorted, distressed look. The brow is more wrinkled, as is the area around the mouth. Eyes may be squeezed shut.

Body Language
1. *Relaxed* is characterized by a calm, restful, mellow appearance. The person seems to be taking it easy.
2. *Tense* is characterized by a strained, apprehensive, or worried appearance. The jaw may be clenched. (Exclude any contractures.)
3. *Distressed pacing* is characterized by activity that seems unsettled. There may be a fearful, worried, or disturbed element present. The rate may be faster or slower.
4. *Fidgeting* is characterized by restless movement. Squirming about or wiggling in the chair may occur. The person might be hitching a chair across the room. Repetitive touching, tugging, or rubbing body parts can also be observed.
5. *Rigid* is characterized by stiffening of the body. The arms and/or legs are tight and inflexible. The trunk may appear straight and unyielding. (Exclude any contractures.)
6. *Fists clenched* is characterized by tightly closed hands. They may be opened and closed repeatedly or held tightly shut.
7. *Knees pulled up* is characterized by flexing the legs and drawing the knees up toward the chest. An overall troubled appearance. (Exclude any contractures.)
8. *Pulling or pushing away* is characterized by resistiveness upon approach or to care. The person is trying to escape by yanking or wrenching him- or herself free or shoving you away.
9. *Striking out* is characterized by hitting, kicking, grabbing, punching, biting, or other form of personal assault.

Consolability
1. *No need to console* is characterized by a sense of well-being. The person appears content.
2. *Distracted or reassured by voice or touch* is characterized by a disruption in the behavior when the person is spoken to or touched. The behavior stops during the period of interaction, with no indication that the person is at all distressed.
3. *Unable to console, distract, or reassure* is characterized by the inability to soothe the person or stop a behavior with words or actions. No amount of comforting, verbal or physical, will alleviate the behavior.

Cornell Scale for Depression in Dementia

The scale is designed as a screening tool and is not diagnostic

2 steps:

1. The clinician interviews the resident's caregiver on each of the 19 items of the scale. The caregiver is instructed to base his / her report on observations of the resident's behaviour during the week prior to the interview
2. The clinician briefly interviews the resident

Total time of administration = approximately 30 minutes

For use with moderate to severely impaired elders with dementia

The scale is valuable to demonstrate effectiveness of interventions, especially antidepressant treatment, when it is completed before the intervention and several weeks after.

Scoring:

1. Each question is scored on a two-point scale: 0 = absent; 1 = mild or intermittent; 2 = severe; n / a = unable to evaluate

2. The caregiver is asked to describe the resident's behaviour observed during the week prior to the interview. Two items, "loss of interest" and "lack of energy" require both a disturbance occurring during the week prior to the interview and relatively acute changes in these areas occurring over less than one month. In these 2 items, the caregiver is instructed to report on the resident's behaviour during the week prior to interview, then give the history of the onset of changes in these 2 areas that may have taken place at an earlier item.

3. The item "suicide" is rated with a score of "1" if the resident has passive suicidal ideation, e.g. feels life is not worth living. A score of "2" is given to subjects who have active suicidal wishes, or have made a recent suicide attempt. History of a suicide attempt in a subject with no passive or active suicidal ideation does not in itself justify a score.

4. If there is a disagreement between the clinician's impression and the caregiver's report, the caregiver is interviewed again in order to clarify the source of discrepancy.

5. Older persons often have disabilities or medical illnesses with symptoms and signs similar to those of depression. Scoring of the Cornell scale on items as "multiple physical complaints", "appetite loss", "weight loss", "lack of energy", and possibly others may be confounded by disability or physical disorder.

   To minimize assignment of falsely high Cornell scale scores in disabled or medically ill residents, raters are instructed to assign a score of "0" for symptoms and signs associated with these conditions. In many cases, the relationship between symptomatology and physical disability or illness is obvious. In some residents, this determination cannot be made reliably.

GEROPSYCHIATRIC EDUCATION PROGRAM
VANCOUVER COASTAL HEALTH

Screening Tool: Cornell Scale for Depression in Dementia (CSDD)

Scoring System: a = unable to evaluate
0 = absent
1 = mild or intermittent
2 = severe

Ratings should be based on symptoms and signs occurring during the week prior to interview. No score should be given if symptoms result from physical disability or illness.

A. Mood-Related Signs

1. Anxiety anxious expression, ruminations, worrying	a	0	1	2
2. Sadness sad expression, sad voice, tearfulness	a	0	1	2
3. Lack of reactivity to pleasant events	a	0	1	2
4. Irritability easily annoyed, short-tempered	a	0	1	2

B. Behavioral Disturbance

1. Agitation restlessness, handwringing, hairpulling	a	0	1	2
2. Retardation slow movements, slow speech, slow reactions	a	0	1	2
3. Multiple physical complaints (score 0 if GI symptoms only)	a	0	1	2
4. Loss of interest less involved in usual activities (score only if change occurred acutely, i.e., in less than 1 month)	a	0	1	2

C. Physical Signs

1. Appetite loss eating less than usual	a	0	1	2
2. Weight loss score 2 if greater than 5 lb. in one month	a	0	1	2
3. Lack of energy fatigues easily, unable to sustain activities (score only if change occurred acutely, i.e., in less than 1 month)	a	0	1	2

continued →

D. Cyclic Functions

1. Diurnal variation of mood symptoms worse in the morning	a	0	1	2
2. Difficulty falling asleep later than usual for this individual	a	0	1	2
3. Multiple awakenings during sleep	a	0	1	2
4. Early-morning awakening earlier than usual for this individual	a	0	1	2

E. Ideational Disturbance

1. Suicide feels life is not worth living, has suicidal wishes or makes suicide attempt	a	0	1	2
2. Poor self-esteem self-blame, self-deprecation, feelings of failure	a	0	1	2
3. Pessimism anticipation of the worst	a	0	1	2
4. Mood-congruent delusions delusions of poverty, illness or loss	a	0	1	2

Scoring:

A score >10 probably major depressive episode
A score >18 definite major depressive episode

Hamilton Anxiety Rating Scale (HAM-A)

Below is a list of phrases that describe certain feeling that people have. Rate the patients by finding the answer which best describes the extent to which he/she has these conditions. Select one of the five responses for each of the fourteen questions.

	Not Present	Mild	Moderate	Severe	Very Severe
1. **Anxious Mood** Worries, anticipation of the worst, fearful anticipation, irritability.	○	○	○	○	○
2. **Tension** Feelings of tension, fatigability, startle response, moved to tears easily, trembling, feelings of restlessness, inability to relax.	○	○	○	○	○
3. **Fears** Of dark, of strangers, of being left alone, of animals, of traffic, of crowds.	○	○	○	○	○
4. **Insomnia** Difficulty in falling asleep, broken sleep, unsatisfying sleep and fatigue on waking, dreams, nightmares, night terrors.	○	○	○	○	○
5. **Intellectual** Difficulty in concentration, poor memory.	○	○	○	○	○
6. **Depressed Mood** Loss of interest, lack of pleasure in hobbies, depression, early waking, diurnal swing.	○	○	○	○	○
7. **Somatic (muscular)** Pains and aches, twitching, stiffness, myoclonic jerks, grinding of teeth, unsteady voice, increased muscular tone.	○	○	○	○	○
8. **Somatic (sensory)** Tinnitus, blurring of vision, hot and cold flushes, feelings of weakness, pricking sensation.	○	○	○	○	○
9. **Cardiovascular Symptoms** Tachycardia, palpitations, pain in chest, throbbing of vessels, fainting feelings, missing beat.	○	○	○	○	○
10. **Respiratory Symptoms** Pressure or constriction in chest, choking feelings, sighing, dyspnea.	○	○	○	○	○
11. **Gastrointestinal Symptoms** Difficulty in swallowing, wind abdominal pain, burning sensations, abdominal fullness, nausea, vomiting, borborygmi, looseness of bowels, loss of weight, constipation.	○	○	○	○	○
12. **Genitourinary Symptoms** Frequency of micturition, urgency of micturition, amenorrhea, menorrhagia, development of rigidity, premature ejaculation, loss of libido, impotence.	○	○	○	○	○
13. **Autonomic Symptoms** Dry mouth, flushing, pallor, tendency to sweat, giddiness, tension headache, raising of hair.	○	○	○	○	○
14. **Behavior at Interview** Fidgeting, restlessness or pacing, tremor of hands, furrowed brow, strained face, sighing or rapid respiration, facial pallor, swallowing, etc.	○	○	○	○	○

THE BRISTOL ACTIVITIES OF DAILY LIVING SCALE (BADLs) EP TEST

1. FOOD
a. Selects and prepares food as required [ ]0
b. Able to prepare food if ingredients set out [ ]1
c. Can prepare food if prompted step by step [ ]2
d. Unable to prep food even w/ prompt & sup [ ]3
e. Not applicable [ ]4

2. EATING
a. Eats appropriately using correct cutlery [ ]0
b. Eats appropriately if food made manageable and/or uses spoon [ ]1
c. Uses fingers to eat [ ]2
d. Needs to be fed [ ]3
e. Not applicable [ ]4

3. DRINK
a. Selects and prepares drinks as required [ ]0
b. Can prepare drinks if ingredients made avail [ ]1
c. Can prep drinks if prompted step by step [ ]2
d. Unable to make drink even w/ prompt/sup [ ]3
e. Not applicable [ ]4

4. DRINKING
a. Drinks appropriately [ ]0
b. Drinks appropriately w/ aids, beaker/straw [ ]1
c. Does not drink appropriately even with aids but attempts to [ ]2
d. Has to have drinks administered (fed) [ ]3
e. Not applicable [ ]4

5. DRESSING
a. Selects appropriate clothing & dresses self [ ]0
b. Puts clothes on in wrong order and/or back to front and or dirty clothing [ ]1
c. Unable to dress self, but moves limbs to assist [ ]2
d. Unable to assist and requires total dsg [ ]3
e. Not applicable [ ]4

6. HYGIENE
a. Washes regularly and independently [ ]0
b. Can wash self if given soap, towel, etc [ ]1
c. Can wash self if prompted and supervised [ ]2
d. Unable to wash self and needs full assist [ ]3
e. Not applicable [ ]4

7. TEETH
a. Cleans own teeth/dentures regularly and I [ ]0
b. Cleans teeth/dentures if given approp items [ ]1
c. Requires some assist, toothpaste on brush [ ]2
d. Full assistance given [ ]3
e. Not applicable [ ]4

8. BATH/SHOWER
a. Bathes regularly and independently [ ]0
b. Needs bath to be drawn/shower turned on but washes independently [ ]1
c. Needs supervision and prompting to wash [ ]2
d. Total dependent, needs supervision [ ]3
e. Not applicable [ ]4

9. TOILET/COMMODE
a. Uses toilet appropriately when required [ ]0
b. Needs to be taken to toilet, & given assist [ ]1
c. Incontinent of urine or feces [ ]2
d. Incontinent of urine and feces [ ]3
e. Not applicable [ ]4

10. TRANSFERS
a. Can get in/out of chair unaided [ ]0
b. Can get in chair but needs help to get out [ ]1
c. Needs help getting in and out of a chair [ ]2
d. Totally dependent on being put into and lifted from a chair [ ]3
e. Not applicable [ ]4

11. MOBILITY
a. Walks independently [ ]0
b. Walks w/assist, ie. furniture, arm for support [ ]1
c. Uses aid to mobilize, ie. frame, stick, etc [ ]2
d. Unable to walk [ ]3
e. Not applicable [ ]4

THE BRISTOL ACTIVITIES OF DAILY LIVING SCALE (BADLs) EP TEST

12. ORIENTATION-TIME
a. Fully orientated to time/day/date etc. [ ]0
b. Unaware of time/day etc. but seems unconcerned [ ]1
c. Repeatedly ask the time/day/date [ ]2
d. Mixes up night and day [ ]3
e. Not applicable [ ]4

13. ORIENTATION-SPACE
a. Fully oriented to surroundings [ ]0
b. Oriented to familiar surroundings only [ ]1
c. Gets lost in home, needs reminding where bathroom is, etc. [ ]2
d. Does not recognize home as own and attempts to leave [ ]3
e. Not applicable [ ]4

14. COMMUNICATION
a. Able to hold appropriate conversation [ ]0
b. Shows understanding and attempts to respond verbally with gestures [ ]1
c. Can make self understood but difficulty understanding others [ ]2
d. Does not respond to or communicate with others [ ]3
e. Not applicable [ ]4

15. TELEPHONE
a. Uses telephone appropriately, including obtaining correct number [ ]0
b. Uses telephone if number given verbally visually or pre-dialed [ ]1
c. Answers telephone but doesn't make calls [ ]2
d. Unable/unwilling to use telephone at all [ ]3
e. Not applicable [ ]4

16. HOUSEWORK/GARDENING
a. Able to do housework/gardening to previous standard [ ]0
b. Able to do housework/gardening but not to previous standard [ ]1
c. Limited participation even with a lot of sup [ ]2
d. Unwilling unable to participate in previous activities [ ]3
e. Not applicable [ ]4

17. SHOPPING
a. Shops to previous standards [ ]0
b. Only able to shop for 1- 2 items w/ or w/o a list [ ]1
c. Unable to shop alone, but participates when accompanied [ ]2
d. Unable to participate in shopping even when accompanied [ ]3
e. Not applicable ` [ ]4

18. FINANCES
a. Responsible for own finances at prev level [ ]0
b. Unable to write check but can sign name and recognizes money value [ ]1
c. Can sign name but unable to recognize money value [ ]2
d. Unable to sign name or recognize money value [ ]3
e. Not applicable [ ]4

19. GAMES/HOBBIES
a. Participate in pastimes/activities to previous standards [ ]0
b. Participates but needs instruction/supervision [ ]1
c. Reluctant to join in, very slow, needs coaxing [ ]2
d. No longer able or willing to join in [ ]3
e. Not applicable [ ]4

TOTAL SCORE: _____

0 = totally independent 60 = totally dependent

© 2022 Tam Cummings, Ph.D. tamcummings.com

VAMC
SLUMS Examination

Questions about this assessment tool? E-mail aging@slu.edu

Name_____ Age_____

Is the patient alert?_____ Level of education_____

___/1 **1** 1. What day of the week is it?

___/1 **1** 2. What is the year?

___/1 **1** 3. What state are we in?

        4. Please remember these five objects. I will ask you what they are later.
          Apple   Pen   Tie   House   Car

        5. You have $100 and you go to the store and buy a dozen apples for $3 and a tricycle for $20.
___/3 **1**   How much did you spend?
      2   How much do you have left?

        6. Please name as many animals as you can in one minute.
___/3   **0** 0-4 animals   **1** 5-9 animals   **2** 10-14 animals   **3** 15+ animals

___/5 7. What were the five objects I asked you to remember? 1 point for each one correct.

        8. I am going to give you a series of numbers and I would like you to give them to me
          backwards. For example, if I say 42, you would say 24.
___/2   **0** 87   **1** 648   **1** 8537

        9. This is a clock face. Please put in the hour markers and the time at
          ten minutes to eleven o'clock.
___/4 **2** Hour markers okay
      2 Time correct

      1 10. Please place an X in the triangle.

___/2 **1** Which of the above figures is largest?

        11. I am going to tell you a story. Please listen carefully because afterwards, I'm going to ask
          you some questions about it.
          Jill was a very successful stockbroker. She made a lot of money on the stock market. She then
          met Jack, a devastatingly handsome man. She married him and had three children. They lived
          in Chicago. She then stopped work and stayed at home to bring up her children. When they were
          teenagers, she went back to work. She and Jack lived happily ever after.
___/8 **2** What was the female's name?   **2** What work did she do?
      2 When did she go back to work?   **2** What state did she live in?

_____ TOTAL SCORE

SCORING

High School Education		Less than High School Education
27-30	Normal	25-30
21-26	Mild Neurocognitive Disorder	20-24
1-20	Dementia	1-19

_____   _____   _____
CLINICIAN'S SIGNATURE   DATE   TIME

SH Tariq, N Tumosa, JT Chibnall, HM Perry III, and JE Morley. The Saint Louis University Mental Status (SLUMS) Examination for detecting mild cognitive impairment and dementia is more sensitive than the Mini-Mental Status Examination (MMSE) - A pilot study. *Am J Geriatr Psych* 14:900-10, 2006.

© 2022 Tam Cummings, Ph.D. tamcummings.com

Short Form of the Informant Questionnaire on Cognitive Decline in the Elderly (Short IQCODE)

Now we want you to remember what your friend or relative was like 10 years ago and to compare it with what he/she is like now. 10 years ago was in 20___.* Below are situations where this person has to use his/her memory or intelligence and we want you to indicate whether this has improved, stayed the same or got worse in that situation over the past 10 years. Note the importance of comparing his/her present performance <u>with 10 years ago</u>. So if 10 years ago this person always forgot where he/she had left things, and he/she still does, then this would be considered "Hasn't changed much". Please indicate the changes you have observed by <u>circling the appropriate answer</u>.

<u>Compared with 10 years ago</u> how is this person at:

	1	2	3	4	5
1. Remembering things about family and friends e.g. occupations, birthdays, addresses	Much improved	A bit improved	Not much change	A bit worse	Much worse
2. Remembering things that have happened recently	Much improved	A bit improved	Not much change	A bit worse	Much worse
3. Recalling conversations a few days later	Much improved	A bit improved	Not much change	A bit worse	Much worse
4. Remembering his/her address and telephone number	Much improved	A bit improved	Not much change	A bit worse	Much worse
5. Remembering what day and month it is	Much improved	A bit improved	Not much change	A bit worse	Much worse
6. Remembering where things are usually kept	Much improved	A bit improved	Not much change	A bit worse	Much worse
7. Remembering where to find things which have been put in a different place from usual	Much improved	A bit improved	Not much change	A bit worse	Much worse
8. Knowing how to work familiar machines around the house	Much improved	A bit improved	Not much change	A bit worse	Much worse

9. Learning to use a new gadget or machine around the house	Much improved	A bit improved	Not much change	A bit worse	Much worse
10. Learning new things in general	Much improved	A bit improved	Not much change	A bit worse	Much worse
11. Following a story in a book or on TV	Much improved	A bit improved	Not much change	A bit worse	Much worse
12. Making decisions on everyday matters	Much improved	A bit improved	Not much change	A bit worse	Much worse
13. Handling money for shopping	Much improved	A bit improved	Not much change	A bit worse	Much worse
14. Handling financial matters e.g. the pension, dealing with the bank	Much improved	A bit improved	Not much change	A bit worse	Much worse
15. Handling other everyday arithmetic problems e.g. knowing how much food to buy, knowing how long between visits from family or friends	Much improved	A bit improved	Not much change	A bit worse	Much worse
16. Using his/her intelligence to understand what's going on and to reason things through	Much improved	A bit improved	Not much change	A bit worse	Much worse

by A. F. Jorm

Centre for Mental Health Research

The Australian National University

Canberra, Australia

The Zarit Burden Interview

0 - NEVER
1 - RARELY
2 - SOMETIMES
3 - QUITE FREQUENTLY
4 - NEARLY ALWAYS

Please circle the response that best describes how you feel.

Question	Score
1 Do you feel that your relative asks for more help than he/she needs?	0 1 2 3 4
2 Do you feel that because of the time you spend with your relative that you don't have enough time for yourself?	0 1 2 3 4
3 Do you feel stressed between caring for your relative and trying to meet other responsibilities for your family or work?	0 1 2 3 4
4 Do you feel embarrassed over your relative's behaviour?	0 1 2 3 4
5 Do you feel angry when you are around your relative?	0 1 2 3 4
6 Do you feel that your relative currently affects our relationships with other family members or friends in a negative way?	0 1 2 3 4
7 Are you afraid what the future holds for your relative?	0 1 2 3 4
8 Do you feel your relative is dependent on you?	0 1 2 3 4
9 Do you feel strained when you are around your relative?	0 1 2 3 4
10 Do you feel your health has suffered because of your involvement with your relative?	0 1 2 3 4
11 Do you feel that you don't have as much privacy as you would like because of your relative?	0 1 2 3 4
12 Do you feel that your social life has suffered because you are caring for your relative?	0 1 2 3 4

Question	Score
13 Do you feel uncomfortable about having friends over because of your relative?	0 1 2 3 4
14 Do you feel that your relative seems to expect you to take care of him/her as if you were the only one he/she could depend on?	0 1 2 3 4
15 Do you feel that you don't have enough money to take care of your relative in addition to the rest of your expenses?	0 1 2 3 4
16 Do you feel that you will be unable to take care of your relative much longer?	0 1 2 3 4
17 Do you feel you have lost control of your life since your relative's illness?	0 1 2 3 4
18 Do you wish you could leave the care of your relative to someone else?	0 1 2 3 4
19 Do you feel uncertain about what to do about your relative?	0 1 2 3 4
20 Do you feel you should be doing more for your relative?	0 1 2 3 4
21 Do you feel you could do a better job in caring for your relative?	0 1 2 3 4
22 Overall, how burdened do you feel in caring for your relative?	0 1 2 3 4

Interpretation of Score:
 0 - 21 little or no burden
21 - 40 mild to moderate burden
41 - 60 moderate to severe burden
61 - 88 severe burden

MM Caregiver Grief Inventory - Short Form

Thomas M. Meuser, Ph.D., University of Missouri – St. Louis
Samuel J. Marwit, Ph.D., University of Missouri-St. Louis (Emeritus)

Instructions: This inventory is designed to measure the grief experience of <u>current</u> family caregivers of persons living with progressive dementia (e.g., Alzheimer's disease). Read each statement carefully, then decide how much you agree or disagree with what is said. Circle a number 1-5 to the right using the answer key below (For example 5 = Strongly Agree). It is important that you respond to all items so that the scores are accurate. Scoring rules are listed below.

ANSWER KEY
1 = Strongly Disagree // 2 = Disagree // 3 = Somewhat Agree // 4 = Agree // 5 = Strongly Agree

#	Statement	1	2	3	4	5	
1	I've had to give up a great deal to be a caregiver.	1	2	3	4	5	A
2	I feel I am losing my freedom.	1	2	3	4	5	A
3	I have nobody to communicate with.	1	2	3	4	5	C
4	I have this empty, sick feeling knowing that my loved one is "gone".	1	2	3	4	5	B
5	I spend a lot of time worrying about the bad things to come.	1	2	3	4	5	C
6	Dementia is like a double loss…I've lost the closeness with my loved one and connectedness with my family.	1	2	3	4	5	C
7	My friends simply don't understand what I'm going through.	1	2	3	4	5	C
8	I long for what was, what we had and shared in the past.	1	2	3	4	5	B
9	I could deal with other serious disabilities better than with this.	1	2	3	4	5	B
10	I will be tied up with this for who knows how long.	1	2	3	4	5	A
11	It hurts to put her/him to bed at night and realize that she/he is "gone"	1	2	3	4	5	B
12	I feel very sad about what this disease has done.	1	2	3	4	5	B
13	I lay awake most nights worrying about what's happening and how I'll manage tomorrow.	1	2	3	4	5	C
14	The people closest to me do not understand what I'm going through.	1	2	3	4	5	C
15	I've lost other people close to me, but the losses I'm experiencing now are much more troubling.	1	2	3	4	5	B
16	Independence is what I've lost…I don't have the freedom to go and do what I want.	1	2	3	4	5	A
17	I wish I had an hour or two to myself each day to pursue personal interests.	1	2	3	4	5	A
18	I'm stuck in this caregiving world and there's nothing I can do about it.	1	2	3	4	5	A

Self-Scoring Procedure: Add the numbers you circled to derive the following sub-scale and total grief scores. Use the letters to the right of each score to guide you.

Personal Sacrifice Burden (A Items) = _____
(6 Items, M = 20.2, SD = 5.3, Alpha = .83, n = 292)

Heartfelt Sadness & Longing (B Items) = _____
(6 Items, M = 20.2, SD = 5.0, Alpha = .80, n = 292)

Worry & Felt Isolation (C Items) = _____
(6 Items, M = 16.6, SD = 5.2, Alpha = .80, n = 292)

Total Grief Level (Sum A + B + C) = _____
(18 Items, M = 57, SD = 12.9, Alpha = .90, n = 292)

Plot your scores using the grid to the right. Make an "**X**" nearest to your numeric score for each sub-scale heading. Connect the X's. This is your grief profile. Discuss this with your support group leader or counselor.

Author Note: This scale may be copied and freely used for clinical or supportive purposes. Those wishing to use the scale for research are asked to e-mail for permission: **meusert@umsl.edu** (8/09).

MM-CGI-SF Personal Grief Profile

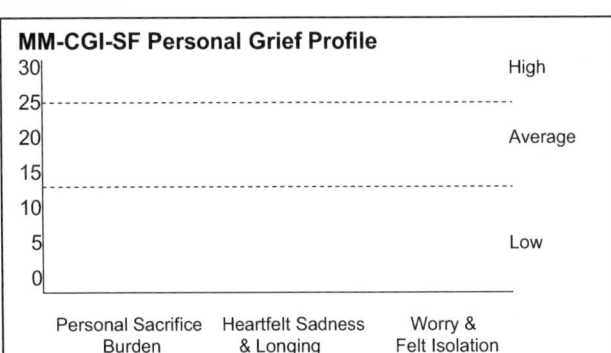

What do these scores mean?
Scores in the top area are one standard deviation (SD) higher than average based on responses of other family caregivers (n = 292). High scores may indicate a need for formal intervention or support assistance to enhance coping. Low scores (one SD below the mean) may indicate denial or a downplaying of distress. Low scores may also indicate positive adaptation if the individual is not showing other signs of suppressed grief or psychological disturbance. Average scores in the center indicate common reactions. These are general guides for discussion and support only— more research is needed on specific interpretation issues.

Geriatric Depression Scale (short form)

Instructions: Circle the answer that best describes how you felt over the <u>past week</u>.

1. Are you basically satisfied with your life?   yes   no
2. Have you dropped many of your activities and interests?   yes   no
3. Do you feel that your life is empty?   yes   no
4. Do you often get bored?   yes   no
5. Are you in good spirits most of the time?   yes   no
6. Are you afraid that something bad is going to happen to you?   yes   no
7. Do you feel happy most of the time?   yes   no
8. Do you often feel helpless?   yes   no
9. Do you prefer to stay at home, rather than going out and doing things?   yes   no
10. Do you feel that you have more problems with memory than most?   yes   no
11. Do you think it is wonderful to be alive now?   yes   no
12. Do you feel worthless the way you are now?   yes   no
13. Do you feel full of energy?   yes   no
14. Do you feel that your situation is hopeless?   yes   no
15. Do you think that most people are better off than you are?   yes   no

Total Score _____

© 2022 Tam Cummings, Ph.D. tamcummings.com

Geriatric Depression Scale (GDS) Scoring Instructions

Instructions: Score 1 point for each bolded answer. A score of 5 or more suggests depression.

1. Are you basically satisfied with your life?   yes   **no**
2. Have you dropped many of your activities and interests?   **yes**   no
3. Do you feel that your life is empty?   **yes**   no
4. Do you often get bored?   **yes**   no
5. Are you in good spirits most of the time?   yes   **no**
6. Are you afraid that something bad is going to happen to you?   **yes**   no
7. Do you feel happy most of the time?   yes   **no**
8. Do you often feel helpless?   **yes**   no
9. Do you prefer to stay at home, rather than going out and doing things?   **yes**   no
10. Do you feel that you have more problems with memory than most?   **yes**   no
11. Do you think it is wonderful to be alive now?   yes   **no**
12. Do you feel worthless the way you are now?   **yes**   no
13. Do you feel full of energy?   yes   **no**
14. Do you feel that your situation is hopeless?   **yes**   no
15. Do you think that most people are better off than you are?   **yes**   no

A score of ≥ 5 suggests depression   **Total Score** _____

Ref. Yes average: The use of Rating Depression Series in the Elderly, in Poon (ed.): Clinical Memory Assessment of Older Adults, American Psychological Association, 1986

NAME: _____   DATE: _____
PATIENT ID#: _____   MD: _____

BRIEF PSYCHIATRIC RATING SCALE (BPRS)

Please enter the score for the term which best describes the patient's condition.

0 = not assessed, 1 = not present, 2 = very mild, 3 = mild, 4 = moderate, 5 = moderately severe, 6 = severe, 7 = extremely severe

1.	**SOMATIC CONCERN** — Degree of concern over present bodily health. Rate the degree to which physical health is perceived as a problem by the patient, whether complaints have a realistic basis or not. SCORE ☐	10.	**HOSTILITY** — Animosity, contempt, belligerence, disdain for other people outside the interview situation. Rate solely on the basis of the verbal report of feelings and actions of the patient toward others; do not infer hostility from neurotic defenses, anxiety, nor somatic complaints. (*Rate attitude toward interviewer under "uncooperativeness"*). SCORE ☐
2.	**ANXIETY** — Worry, fear, or over-concern for present or future. Rate solely on the basis of verbal report of patient's own subjective experiences. Do not infer anxiety from physical signs or from neurotic defense mechanisms. SCORE ☐	11.	**SUSPICIOUSNESS** — Brief (*delusional or otherwise*) that others have now, or have had in the past, malicious or discriminatory intent toward the patient. On the basis of verbal report, rate only those suspicions which are currently held whether they concern past or present circumstances. SCORE ☐
3.	**EMOTIONAL WITHDRAWAL** — Deficiency in relating to the interviewer and to the interviewer situation. Rate only the degree to which the patient gives the impression of failing to be in emotional contact with other people in the interview situation. SCORE ☐	12.	**HALLUCINATORY BEHAVIOR** — Perceptions without normal external stimulus correspondence. Rate only those experiences which are reported to have occurred within the last week and which are described as distinctly different from the thought and imagery processes of normal people. SCORE ☐
4.	**CONCEPTUAL DISORGANIZATION** — Degree to which the thought processes are confused, disconnected, or disorganized. Rate on the basis of integration of the verbal products of the patient; do not rate on the basis of patient's subjective impression of his own level of functioning. SCORE ☐	13.	**MOTOR RETARDATION** — Reduction in energy level evidenced in slowed movements. Rate on the basis of observed behavior of the patient only; do not rate on the basis of patient's subjective impression of own energy level. SCORE ☐
5.	**GUILT FEELINGS** — Over-concern or remorse for past behavior. Rate on the basis of the patient's subjective experiences of guilt as evidenced by verbal report with appropriate affect; do not infer guilt feelings from depression, anxiety or neurotic defenses. SCORE ☐	14.	**UNCOOPERATIVENESS** — Evidence of resistance, unfriendliness, resentment, and lack of readiness to cooperate with the interviewer. Rate only on the basis of the patient's attitude and responses to the interviewer and the interview situation; do not rate on basis of reported resentment or uncooperativeness outside the interview situation. SCORE ☐
6.	**TENSION** — Physical and motor manifestations of tension "nervousness", and heightened activation level. Tension should be rated solely on the basis of physical signs and motor behavior and not on the basis of subjective experiences of tension reported by the patient. SCORE ☐	15.	**UNUSUAL THOUGHT CONTENT** — Unusual, odd, strange or bizarre thought content. Rate here the degree of unusualness, not the degree of disorganization of thought processes. SCORE ☐
7.	**MANNERISMS AND POSTURING** — Unusual and unnatural motor benavior, the type of motor behavior which causes certain mental patients to stand out in a crowd of normal people. Rate only abnormality of movements; do not rate simple heightened motor activity here. SCORE ☐	16.	**BLUNTED AFFECT** — Reduced emotional tone, apparent lack of normal feeling or involvement. SCORE ☐
8.	**GRANDIOSITY** — Exaggerated self-opinion, conviction of unusual ability or powers. Rate only on the basis of patient's statements about himself or self-in-relation-to-others, not on the basis of his demeanor in the interview situation. SCORE ☐	17.	**EXCITEMENT** — Heightened emotional tone, agitation, increased reactivity. SCORE ☐
9.	**DEPRESSIVE MOOD** — Despondency in mood, sadness. Rate only degree of despondency; do not rate on the basis of inferences concerning depression based upon general retardation and somatic complaints. SCORE ☐	18.	**DISORIENTATION** — Confusion or lack of proper association for person, place or time. SCORE ☐

© 2022 Tam Cummings, Ph.D. tamcummings.com

Additional Books & Resources
by Dr. Tam Cummings

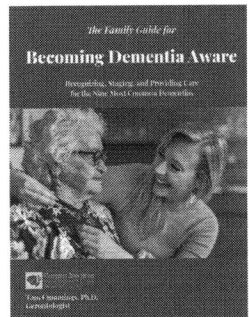

Becoming Dementia Aware — *the Family Guide*
Designed especially for family caregivers, this fully illustrated book will help you understand the causes and behaviors associated with dementia and offers tips for improving care and coping with the stress of providing care.

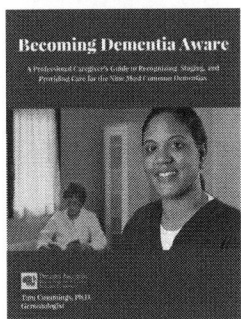

Becoming Dementia Aware — *the Guide for Professionals*
Designed especially for professional caregivers to accompany *Becoming Dementia Aware* training. It's a complete, fully illustrated resource for virtually every aspect of the nine most common forms of dementia.

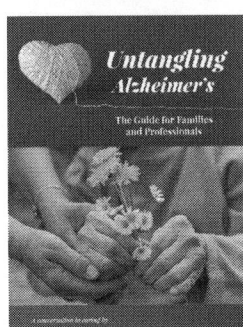

Untangling Alzheimer's
Dr. Cummings provides all you need to know about dementia in this indispensable guide for family members and professional caregivers. Comprehensive, yet highly readable, it helps family members and caregivers understand the causes and behaviors associated with the nine most common forms of dementia, what to expect, and how to provide better care.

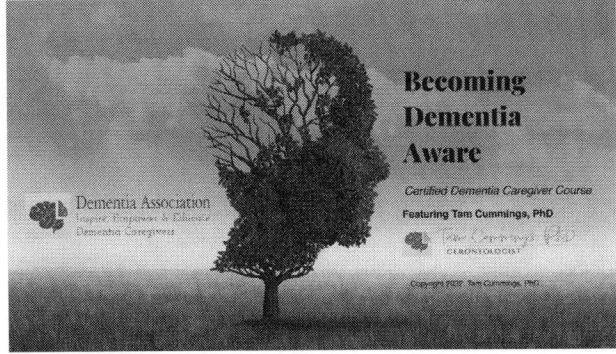

Becoming Dementia Aware Videos

Videos that provide a complete understanding of the 7 stages of dementia, the symptoms of each and what to expect in behaviors—and how to provide better care at each stage of the disease.

Dr. Cummings provides on-site training for professional caregivers, but memory care communities can access the same training at a greatly reduced cost through her video training series. Videos for family caregivers are also available. For more information, visit **https://www.tamcummings.com**.

For additional information on Dr. Cummings, visit https://www.tamcummings.com.

Made in the USA
Columbia, SC
18 June 2025

59573020R00078